The Mediterranean Diet For Beginners

Lose Weight and Eat Healthily

Jenny De Luca

Copyright © 2014 Jenny De Luca

All rights reserved.

DEDICATION

This book is dedicated to my family for the inspiration they provide me every day.

CONTENTS

Introduction 1
What Is The Mediterranean Diet? 3
How The Mediterranean Diet Benefits You 5
Stocking Your Cupboards 7
Mediterranean Breakfast REcipes 9
Mediterranean Lunch Recipes 21
Mediterranean Dinner Recipes 35
Mediterranean Dessert Recipes 50
Mediterranean Snack REcipes 60
Mediterranean Bread Recipes 68
The Mediterranean Diet On A Budget 78
What To Eat And What To Avoid 80
The Importance Of WIne In This Diet 84
Loosing Weight By Eating Mediterranean 86
7 Day Mediterranean Diet PLan 88
Mediterranean Diet Tips 90
Endnote 93

ACKNOWLEDGMENTS

The people of the Mediterranean for eating in such a healthy way that can benefit us all plus my family for being such an inspiration to find and follow this diet.

INTRODUCTION

In Western countries, from America to the Western parts of Europe, the health of the population is in decline and whilst longevity is improving often it is at the cost of quality of life. One in every four deaths in the USA is due to heart disease, which is one of the diseases that the Mediterranean Diet minimizes the risk of.

The rise of the various health problems can be linked directly to the decrease in the quality of diet and the increase in artificial and processed foods consumed by the popular. In areas which still eat a more natural diet, diseases such as cancer, diabetes and heart disease are significantly lower, so much so that scientists are investigating the contributing health factors from this diet.

Two of the biggest killers in America are cardiovascular disease (over a million lives a year) and cancer. According to the American Cancer Society in a 2005 report at least half of the cancer related deaths could be prevented if Americans took care of their health by eating better and exercising more. The store is much the same in the United Kingdom and rapidly becoming the same in Western Europe too, yet is completely different in areas which follow the Mediterranean Diet.

Obesity is being hailed as a major crisis for our generation with well over 60% of people in the West being overweight which increases the risk of diabetes, high blood pressure and many other problems. Yet in countries that follow the Mediterranean Diet, these problems are incredibly rare and the people enjoy a long, productive life!

Whilst it is impossible at present to wipe out these problems it is possible to minimize the risk of them and do your best to prevent them just by making some changes to your diet and increasing your level of exercise. You do not have to spend hours every day at the gym, but some simple changes to your lifestyle will make your risk of developing these diseases plummet.

The Mediterranean Diet focusses heavily on healthy, fresh foods with very few, if any, processed high sugar foods that many Westerners rely on. The diet uses healthy oils that actually benefit you rather than the dangerous oils used in much of our cooking.

Current research is showing just how beneficial the Mediterranean Diet is for you. The combination of healthy olive oil, nuts, avocados and vegetables work together to create nitro fatty acids which lower your blood pressure. The unsaturated fat in the oil works with the nitrites in the other components to benefit your health! These nitro fatty acids then block an enzyme called epoxide hydrolase which causes your blood pressure to decrease.

This book will help you to understand what the Mediterranean Diet is and how you can benefit from it. It contains plenty of recipes that are affordable and easy to make which are not only healthy for you but taste fantastic too! These come from countries in the Mediterranean area including Italy, Greece and Lebanon; all of which eat this healthy diet and reap the benefits of it.

The nice thing about this diet is it is not one where you feel you have to struggle with what to eat or have to go without the foods you like. The diet is full of delicious, nutritious and tasty meals that are an absolutely pleasure to eat! The entire diet is focused on good quality nutrition that is full of vitamins and minerals that help your body to heal and repair itself.

In order for you to really make the most of this diet you will need to make a few small changes to your lifestyle. Follow the eating plans and change your diet so you are eating this nutritious food. Take a 20 to 30 minute walk every day and make sure there is time in your calendar for relaxation and recuperation. Finally, make sure you get a good eight hours of good quality sleep every night. I know this last one is not possible for all of us due to children or working patterns, but do your best as sleep is vital to your health; it's when the body heals itself!

The biggest difference between the typical American diet, which is very convenient, and the Mediterranean Diet is that the former is full of over-processed, artificial foods, vegetables and grains that are cooked in such a way as to remove most of the nutrition. It really is a health hazard and should carry a warning label!

On the island of Ikaria residents follow the Mediterranean lifestyle. They eat good quality food, enjoy locally produced wine most days, exercise in moderation and spend time with their friends and family relaxing and enjoying their company. The result is a very healthy population who are active and healthy well into their 90's with many living to be over 100 years old!

The Nuoro province of Sardinia has the highest concentration of male centenarians in the world, and they follow the Mediterranean diet. Okinawa has the longest lived women in the world and they too follow a very similar diet to the Mediterranean people.

At the end of the day, the Mediterranean diet is going to make you feel healthier, live longer and reduce your risk of disease and illness. This book has been written to help you to understand the diet and give you some great ideas for food you can eat. I know from my own experience that this diet is full of delicious food and that I do not miss the stodgy, heavy, overly processed foods. Once your taste buds adjust to eating more fresh food you will really be able to notice how terrible the food you ate previously tastes as the fresh and wholesome food on this diet is truly delicious.

The aim of the book is not to preach to you but to show you how this diet can benefit you and your family. When you follow this diet and eat well you are going to see some major benefits to your health and by reducing your calorie intake through this diet you will also lose weight.

You deserve to give yourself the best in life and I know from my own personal point of view I want to stay healthy for as long as possible so I can enjoy my children and see my grandchildren. Living a long time is one thing, but quality of life is the most important thing; for those on the island if Ikaria they are tending vineyards, walking around and active into their 90's and beyond.

Enjoy this book and try the recipes in it. As you get used to cooking in this fashion, try branching out and experimenting, but most of all enjoy eating in this healthy and beneficial manner.

WHAT IS THE MEDITERRANEAN DIET?

The Mediterranean Diet refers to a specific diet eaten by people who live in the countries on the shores of the Mediterranean Sea including Italy, Greek, Lebanon and so on. The diet does not mean you have to eat foods from those countries, but instead recommends the types of food you should eat. It refers to a diet and a lifestyle which promotes good health and longevity.

This diet includes a wide variety of food, including high levels of fresh fruit and vegetables which give your body all the vitamins, minerals and other nutrients it needs to heal and repair itself. Because much of the food consumed in these areas is locally grown they also eat foods which are available in season though you will have access to fresh fruits and vegetables all year round from the supermarket.

The Western diet is very high in salt, with it added to many meals and virtually all fast foods, which increases your blood pressure and has been proven to be bad for your health. The Mediterranean people do not rely on salt for their flavoring but instead use herbs which will open up a whole new world of flavor to you!

The Mediterranean Diet is not about super foods and quick fixes and is not really a strict list, more a set of guidelines of what will help you to be a healthier person. Of course when you go out for a meal or fancy something else you can have it, but the majority of your diet should be these healthy food stuffs.

To give you an idea of what the diet involves, these guidelines will help you to understand the Mediterranean Diet.

- High intake of vegetables, legumes, fruits and wholegrain cereals.
- Limited intake of red meat substituting poultry and fish instead.
- Olive oil or rapeseed oil are used instead of animal fats like lard or butter. These mono-unsaturated fats are very healthy and beneficial for you.
- Processed and fast foods are avoided as are ready meals as these are high in preservatives, fats and salt.
- Dairy is eaten but in a moderate amount, typically low fat versions.
- Salt is not added to the food at the table as there is plenty already in the meal.
- Snacks consist of fruit, unsalted nuts and dried fruit.
- Red wine is drunk with meals and typical intake is just two or three glasses per day.
- Water is the best drink to have instead of soda and other sugary drinks. Tea and

coffee in moderation can be beneficial too.

The Mediterranean Diet is a great way to eat if you want to improve your health and energy levels. It has been proven to be highly effective and more and more people are turning to this revolutionary way of living which is making a huge difference to its followers.

It is not a hard diet to follow but is a very enjoyable diet enjoyed by people across the Mediterranean basin. Many people in the West are discovering this diet and with the focus from scientists on this diet and how it benefits people, it is only going to become more and more popular. It is a surprisingly easy diet to eat and very enjoyable. Unlike specific weight loss diets you are never going without and have a wide variety of delicious foods to eat.

By substituting the highly processed, high sugar, high fat foods that many of us eat with more natural and healthier alternatives you can find that not only do you lose weight, but you also improve your health too and feel fantastic. This book will explain exactly how you can follow the Mediterranean Diet as well as show you how you can easily stick to it and thoroughly enjoy the whole process. With the many benefits you are going to receive from this diet, you will be wanting to start it today as you realize just how much it will benefit you!

HOW THE MEDITERRANEAN DIET BENEFITS YOU

You will have heard people singing the praises of the Mediterranean Diet and are probably wondering what makes it so good. Scientists have invested a lot of time and money in understanding this diet because it contributes to longevity and reduces the risk of many chronic diseases which are rife in the West including Alzheimer's, cancer, diabetes, heart disease and more.

The benefits of this diet were first noticed in the 1970's during a study by the University of Minnesota who realized that heart related diseases and deaths were significantly lower along the Mediterranean basin part of Greece than it was in America and other industrialized nations.

The conclusion of the study was that the good health could be directly attributed to the fact that dietary fat came from vegetables rather than highly saturated fats which come from meat and dairy.

A similar study in 1988 in France (The Lyon Heart Study) showed that the Mediterranean diet significantly reduced the number of heart attacks in the people who followed this diet. In 1990 the World Health Organization showed that the inhabitants of the Mediterranean region were 50% less like to die from heart diseases than people in the United States of America.

As research into this diet continued so the evidence keeps on stacking up for it being a healthy and beneficial way of eating! In 2003 a join study between Athens and Harvard Universities concluded that following the traditional Mediterranean diet is associated with longevity. In 2005 a study by The Lancet concluded that the reduction in consumption of fresh fruit and vegetables was directly linked to the increase in cancer rates.

Time and time again studies have shown that this form of diet is extremely beneficial to your health and longevity plus it is one diet where the food is absolutely delicious and you really do not feel like you are going without! Extra virgin olive oil seems to be a major contributing factor to these benefits as it is a beneficial mono-unsaturated fat which is much healthier than the saturated fats typically consumed in the West.

The Mediterranean Diet places a strong emphasis on consuming leafy green vegetables, cruciferous vegetables and fruits that have high levels of phytochemicals. These include anti-oxidants which stop free radicals damaging your body and reduces the risk of heart disease, cancer and other serious health complaints.

Being on the shores of the Mediterranean it is only natural that this diet should include seafood, which is a great source of Omega-3 fatty acids, also proven to be very beneficial to your health. These can be found in eggs and walnuts too, both of which are eaten on the Mediterranean Diet.

In the West many carbohydrates are bleached and processed, removing most of the goodness from them. In the Mediterranean Diet they are left in a complex state and are highly nutritious.

With the rise of diets such as the Paleo diet which focuses purely on fresh fruit and vegetables, you can see that just eating these will benefit your health, yet for many people diets like the Paleo are too restrictive and too difficult to follow. When following any diet it is important that it fits in with your lifestyle. The Mediterranean Diet offers all the benefits of the Paleo diet and more with delicious, cooked food that fits in to your lifestyle and is relatively easy to prepare.

Diet is the easiest and best way for you to look after your health and reduce the risk of serious or chronic illness. Many people have found that just by changing the way they eat that they have changed their health. This way of eating is working for people across the world, including the original followers of the diet. It is a natural way of eating that has been proven time and time again to have massive benefits to your health and wellness.

Scientists are concluding that the Mediterranean Diet has significant health benefits to the people who follow it. It is a very easy diet to follow and is surprisingly tasty and good fun! For anyone who wants to improve their health and reduce their risk of diseases this is a diet you should be following.

STOCKING YOUR CUPBOARDS

Shopping when you are following the Mediterranean diet is slightly different from shopping on the usual Western diet. Before we head in to the recipes and start talking about the delicious dishes you can cook you need to know a little bit about the staples that you will have in your cupboards for these recipes and more.

On the Western diet a lot of meat is typically eaten. Usually it is fatty red meat which is not good for you at all and usually it has salt or other chemicals added and is cooked in yet more unhealthy fats! Red meat is not eaten very often on the Mediterranean Diet with fish and poultry being consumed more frequently.

Oily fish such as sardines and anchovies are often eaten as they are very high in Omega-3 oils, which are excellent for your body. Other seafood such as salmon, mussels, shrimp, halibut and flounder are all eaten. Poultry of all sorts is another essential source of lean protein as are eggs. Other protein sources include walnuts, tofu, tempeh, unsalted almonds and walnuts, lentils, beans and other legumes are all eaten. There are a variety for sale in your local supermarket though try to avoid any that have been processed or have had additives added to them.

Dairy products feature in the Mediterranean Diet and often this comes from sheep or goats milk, e.g. feta cheese rather than our Western cow's milk cheeses. This is a less processed and more natural cheese that is much healthier for you. Low fat yogurt, sour cream and milk can all be eaten as can milk alternatives such as soy, almond, hemp and rice milk all make for delicious alternatives to dairy milk that are very good for you.

Cereals such as steel cut oatmeal and unsweetened shredded wheat are eaten but the sugary, chemical laden cereals eaten in the west are avoided.

Spices feature heavily in Mediterranean cooking and are the main source of flavor. Salt is rarely used and if it is then it is usually sea salt. Herbs can be used fresh or dried. Dill, basil, parsley, oregano and thyme are all firm favorites and garlic (a miracle food in itself) features heavily as a flavoring. Lemon and lime make for a piquant addition to dishes and balsamic vinegar gives it a tang. Mustard, horseradish and capers are all popular seasonings in this style of cooking.

Only extra-virgin olive oil is used, nothing more as it is extremely good for you and is great on salads, bread and more. It can be used in virtually any cooking and is great for your heart!

Breads and pasta feature very heavily in the Mediterranean Diet but they tend to be wholegrain versions and not the bleached and processed white versions eaten in the West.

The white versions tend to be devoid of nutrition and the health benefits come from the whole grains used in the bread and pasta. Quinoa, whole grain couscous and brown rice are all a part of this diet and are proven to be extremely healthy and full of vitamins and minerals.

Vegetables are a major part of the Mediterranean Diet and leafy green vegetables are very popular. Tomatoes, peppers, eggplant, onions and more are all a key component, all of which are proving to have various health benefits. One vegetable which is less commonly eaten around the Mediterranean is the potato, though sweet potatoes and squashes are popular.

Fresh fruit also is a major part of the diet with melon (a very alkaline fruit) being one of the main fruits eaten. Grapes, berries, pineapple and mango are all a significant part of this diet and these are all full of goodness that your body really benefits from.

Even the humble avocado is featured in the Mediterranean Diet and it is full of healthy fats. It makes a great addition to a salad and can be made in to guacamole or other dips which can be a nice addition to any meal.

You will also want to stock up on canned tomatoes, beans, chickpeas, kidney beans and so on. All of these need to be low sodium versions and they are very healthy for you containing both proteins and healthy fats as well as plenty of micro-nutrients.

Unsweetened dark chocolate is eaten and wines are drunk, with red wines being particularly favored.

This is a little bit different from the typical American shopping list and it may take you a little while to kick the habit of filling your trolley with unhealthy foods. However, once you get stuck in to it you will soon realize that this diet is good fun, varied and that the foods are absolutely delicious!

MEDITERRANEAN BREAKFAST RECIPES

Breakfast is probably the most important meal of the day, particularly if you want to lose weight. When you eat breakfast you kick start your metabolism for the day and if you skip breakfast your metabolism stays sleepy for the day. Eating a good breakfast helps you to lose weight by setting your body up to burn calories.

The best breakfasts are high in protein and low in sugars. High sugar breakfasts contribute to the risk of diabetes and results in a sugar crash around mid-morning, which ends up with you craving unhealthy snacks. For many people though, breakfast is something that has to happen in a hurry so many of these recipes are quick or can be made in advance.

Yogurt is a great way for you to start your day but be aware that many of the processed yogurts can be very high in sugar. Natural or Greek yogurt is great to use particularly when mixed with the some fresh berries.

Steel cut / whole grain oatmeal is proven to improve the health of your heart and add fiber to your diet. You can make oatmeal with milk, soymilk, almond milk or water depending on your taste and add sweetness with honey, fresh or dried fruit or even maple syrup. Be aware that the instant oatmeals are usually very high in sugar and other synthetics which are not so good for you.

Fruit smoothies are a great way to start the day and can be blended with any type of milk, fruit juice or liquid yogurt. There is a lot of variety possible here and you can tailor the smoothies according to what is in season, affordable and your personal tastes.

Eggs are a very versatile breakfast though preparing them fresh can take some time, which may be difficult if you are in a rush in the morning. However some of the dishes such as frittata's can be made in advance and just heated up. Whether you eat your egg boiled, fried (in olive oil) or scrambled, it can make a great breakfast, particularly when served with some whole grain bread.

There are a lot of options for your breakfast on the Mediterranean Diet and this section will open your eyes and help you to eat well on this diet.

Asparagus And Salmon Omelette

This is an unusual breakfast but one that is very tasty and high in Omega 3, which comes from the salmon and the eggs. It does not take that long to cook and is worth taking the time to make. It can make a nice lunch or be part of a dinner as well if you would like.

Ingredients:
- 4oz fresh salmon (de-boned)
- 2 eggs
- 2 asparagus spears (lightly steamed)
- 1 clove garlic (minced)
- 2 tablespoons diced onion
- ½ tablespoon parsley
- 1 teaspoon lemon juice
- 1 teaspoon low fat milk
- ½ teaspoon olive oil
- Salt / Pepper / Dill / Chives for garnish and to taste

Method:
1. Heat the oil in a non-stick pan over a medium heat and sauté the onions for around three minutes until translucent.
2. Add the garlic, lemon juice and asparagus and cook for another two minutes.
3. In a medium bowl beat the milk and eggs together with the parsley. Season to taste with the herbs.
4. Slowly pour the eggs into the pan ensuring the bottom of the pan is covered and allow to set (around 90 seconds).
5. Sprinkle the salmon over the egg mixture and reduce the heat to a low setting.
6. Allow to cook for around three minutes before folding in half and cooking for another minute.

Cheesy Nutty Toast

This is a quick breakfast that is really tasty and jam packed with essential nutrients to get your body going for the day.

Ingredients:
- 1 slice of whole grain bread
- ¾oz low calorie cheese
- ½ pear (peeled, cored and sliced)
- ½ teaspoon chopped walnuts

Method:
1. Toast the bread and then spread the cheese on it.
2. Top with the walnuts and pear and eat immediately.

Fruity Nutty Granola

This is a nice breakfast that is great for anyone who likes cereal and is very tasty. It incorporates many of the healthy parts of the Mediterranean Diet. Just make sure that you buy a healthy granola, ideally organic without added sugar as otherwise you will be undoing many of the benefits of this eating program.

Ingredients:
- ½ cup granola (low fat no added sugar)
- ½ cup milk (or substitute)
- ¼ sliced banana
- ¼ apple (peeled and diced)
- 1 teaspoon chopped walnuts

Method:
1. Pour the granola in to a bowl and add the milk.
2. Sprinkle the apple, walnuts and banana over the top.

Mediterranean Breakfast Smoothie

Smoothies are a great quick breakfast that provides you with quickly absorbed nutrients. This also makes a good snack for during the day and can be varied by using different berries depending on what is in season and available.

Ingredients:
- 2oz pomegranate juice (pure is best with no added sugar)
- ½ banana
- ½ cup berries (strawberries, raspberries or blueberries or a mixture of these)
- ¼ cup apple juice (no added sugar)
- ½ tablespoon flaxseed
- 5 or 6 ice cubes (to taste)

Method:
1. Add all the ingredients to a blender and blend on a high setting until smooth.
2. Pour in to a tall glass and serve immediately.

Fruit And Nut Oatmeal

Oatmeal is a good breakfast because it is filling and provides energy throughout the morning. With the added fruit and nuts you are getting extra vitamins and minerals that are vital for your health and ensuring you keep going until lunchtime.

Ingredients:
- ½ cup steel rolled oats
- ¼ mango (peeled and diced)
- ½ apple (cored, peeled and diced)
- 1 cup milk (or substitute)
- 1 teaspoon sliced almonds
- 1 teaspoon sunflower seeds

Method:
1. Mix the oats and milk in a microwave proof bowl or in a pan, depending on your preference. Microwave for a couple of minutes.
2. Mix in the sunflower seeds and almonds before topping with the fruit and serving.

Mediterranean Frittata

This is a good, filling breakfast that will serve two people. It takes less than ten minutes to prepare and about the same to cook. It is very healthy and you can vary the ingredients or add more vegetables to make it more substantial if you prefer.

Ingredients:
- 6 eggs
- 4 egg whites
- 2 green onions (finely chopped)
- ¾ cup baby spinach (make sure it is packed then coarsely chop it)
- 1/3 cup feta cheese (this is nice with a basil and sun-dried tomato cheese)
- 2 tablespoons olive oil
- 2 tablespoons Greek seasoning (salt free)
- Dash of salt (optional)

Method:
1. Preheat your broiler or grill.
2. Heat the oil in an over-proof skillet.
3. Meanwhile in a bowl mix the eggs, cheese, seasoning and egg whites and whisk well.
4. Add in the spinach and onion and stir well.
5. Pour the egg mixture into the skillet and cook for around two minutes until the edges are set. Carefully lift the edge of the mixture and tilt the pan so that the uncooked egg mixture comes in to contact with the pan.
6. Cook for a further 2 minutes until the eggs are virtually set.
7. Broil or grill for a couple of minutes until the middle is set.
8. Transfer to a plate and cut in to four wedges

Mediterranean Breakfast Wraps

This breakfast takes around thirty minutes to prepare and cook, so is good for a lazy weekend morning but will serve four. It is very healthy and a great start to the day.

Ingredients:
- 6 eggs
- Flour tortillas
- ¾ cup feta cheese (crumbled)
- ¼ cup sour cream (low fat)
- 2 tablespoons roasted red peppers (diced)
- 2 tablespoons green onions (minced)
- ½ teaspoon each of basil and oregano
- ¼ teaspoon garlic powder

Method:
1. Preheat a skillet on a medium heat
2. In a bowl whisk the cream, eggs and seasonings together.
3. Gently stir in the feta cheese.
4. Add a teaspoon of olive oil to the pan when it is hot and then add the eggs.
5. As the eggs start to set scrape the bottom of the pan to allow the runny parts of the eggs to start to set.
6. Stir in the peppers and onion and cook until it reaches your preferred consistency.
7. Serve immediately wrapped in warmed tortillas and garnished with chives, parsley or crumbled feta cheese.

La Trouchia

This is an omelette from the Nice region in France where it is made with Swiss chard. It is similar to the frittata and a tian, which is found in Provence. This recipe will serve four people and is pleasantly filling.

Ingredients:
- 6 eggs
- 8 black olives
- 1 clove of garlic (minced)
- 1 onion (finely chopped)
- 1lb Swiss chard (remove stems and coarsely shred the leaves)
- 1 cup Parmigianino Reggiano cheese (grated)
- 5 tablespoons olive oil
- 2 tablespoons flat leaf parsley (chopped)

Method:
1. Heat 3 tablespoons of olive oil in a non-stick pan on a medium heat then sauté the onion for around a minute until softened.
2. Add the chard and cook until wilted.
3. Reduce the heat and continue to cook, stirring frequently for a further 6 minutes until tender and then put to one side to cool.
4. In a bowl, beat the eggs until well blended then stir in half the cheese together with all of the parsley and garlic.
5. Season to taste and add the chard mixture, stirring to mix.
6. Wipe the pan out with a paper towel and return to a low heat. Add the rest of the olive oil.
7. Once heated, add the egg mixture, stirring gently. As soon as the eggs begin to set, stop stirring the mixture.
8. Leave the eggs to heat for around 4 minutes then place a plate over the pan. Hold the plate and pan together and turn, lifting the set egg mixture out of the pan. Slip the omelette back in to the pan and return to the heat.
9. Sprinkle the rest of the cheese over the top of the omelette and cook for another 2 to 3 minutes.
10. Slide the omelette on to a serving plate and place the olives on the top. Cut into wedges and serve immediately.

Greek Yogurt Parfaits

This makes an excellent breakfast or dessert and is made from grano which can be found in Italian markets or health food stores. As an alternative you can use brown rice, pearly barley or wheat berries. This recipe will serve 8 people and takes about an hour to make, most of which is cooking the grano.

Ingredients:
- 1 cup grano (uncooked)
- 12 cups of water (divided)
- 4 cups Greek yogurt
- 2 cups berries (fresh is best though frozen and thawed will do)
- ¼ cup orange blossom honey
- ¼ teaspoon salt

Method:
1. Soak the grano overnight in 6 cups of water.
2. Boil the other 6 cups in a medium pan, add the grano then reduce the heat and simmer for around 20 minutes until tender.
3. Drain well then stir in the salt and honey before cooling to room temperature.
4. Spoon a quarter cup of yogurt in to each of 8 parfait glasses and top with 3 tablespoons of grano and 2 tablespoons of berries.
5. Repeat the layers until all of the ingredients are used up.

Middle Eastern Breakfast

This is a very popular dish in the Middle East around the Mediterranean coastline and can include a cucumber salad too. This recipe will serve 4 people and can take almost two hours to make so is not ideal for those mornings when you are in a rush, but is ideal to impress visitors and provide a hearty breakfast before a day out.

Ingredients:
- 2 wholemeal pita breads (cut into 8 wedges each)
- 4 eggs
- 1 cup water
- 1 cup plum tomatoes (chopped and seeded)
- ½ cup fresh parsley (chopped)
- 1/8 cup bulgur wheat (uncooked)
- 4 tablespoons extra virgin olive oil (divided)
- 2 tablespoons lemon juice (fresh is best)
- 2 tablespoons purple onion (finely chopped)
- 1½ tablespoons fresh mint (chopped)
- ½ teaspoon salt (divided)
- Good twist of black pepper
- Dash of ground red pepper

Method:
1. Preheat your oven to 350F.
2. Arrange the pita wedges as a single layer on a baking sheet and lightly brush with 2 tablespoons of olive oil. Bake until golden, which will take around 20 minutes.
3. In a large bowl mix a cup of water together with the bulgur wheat and leave to stand for around 30 minutes until the bulgur is tender.
4. Drain the bulgur thoroughly using a sieve and discard the liquid.
5. Put the bulgur in a medium bowl and add 2 tablespoons of oil plus the parsley, tomato, mint, lemon juice, onion and the seasoning.
6. Toss this mixture well and refrigerate for half an hour.
7. Boil a medium sized saucepan of water and using a slotted spoon put the eggs carefully in the pan.
8. Cook for 6 minutes then drain and rinse the eggs under cold running water for about a minute until cool. Then peel the eggs.
9. Place about a third of a cup of the bulgar mixture (Tabbouleh) on a plate with 4 pita wedges and top with an egg. Sprinkle the eggs with salt, pepper or parsley as required.

Magnificent Mediterranean Muesli

This breakfast dish is popular on the African shores of the Mediterranean and can be stored in the refrigerator for a few days. Avoid instant oatmeal as it is high in artificial sugar. Irish oatmeal or other steel cut oats works well in this dish. It can be made the night before and will serve four people. This will give you plenty of energy throughout the morning and is perfect on a cold winter's day.

Ingredients:
- 1 cup oats
- 1 cup milk (or substitute)
- 1 cup plain yogurt (low fat ideally)
- ¼ cup oat bran
- ¼ cup honey
- ½ cup walnuts (coarsely chopped)
- 2½ teaspoons each of dried fig, dried apricot and pitted date (all chopped)
- Raspberries or other fresh berries (optional)

Method:
1. Mix all the ingredients (except the berries) in a bowl and chill for 2 hours or overnight.
2. Garnish with fresh berries when serving.

Roasted Spiced Pistachio Flavoring

This blend of apricots and pomegranate seeds mixed with warm spices is delicious and can be used to flavor oatmeal, yogurt or muesli. It will really give the breakfast a very warm flavor. This recipe will serve 12 though is so nice you may want to use double in your breakfasts! It can be made up to three days in advance if using fresh fruit and a week if using dried.

Ingredients:

- 1½ cups pistachios (unsalted and roasted)
- ½ cup dried apricots (chopped)
- ¼ cup dried pomegranate seeds (dried cranberries make a good alternative)
- 2 teaspoons sugar
- ½ teaspoon cinnamon
- ¼ teaspoon ground allspice
- ¼ teaspoon ground nutmeg

Method:
1. Preheat your oven to 350F.
2. Spread out the pistachios on a rimmed baking sheet and cook for around 7 minutes until lightly toasted. Remove from oven and cool completely.
3. Toss all the ingredients together in a bowl until well coated.

Poached Eggs – Turkish Style

Eggs are a big part of the Turkish diet and here they are set on a bed of yogurt and drizzled with a red pepper and sage butter, which gives it a bit of a kick. This recipe will serve 4 people and takes around 20 minutes to make. It can be served with home-made hummus (see the snack section) or Tabbouleh (see above).

Ingredients:

- 8 eggs
- 2 garlic cloves (pressed)
- Pita bread (warmed)
- 1 cup plain yogurt
- ¼ cup olive oil (or unsalted butter which is more authentic but unhealthier)
- 1 tablespoon distilled white vinegar
- ½ teaspoon paprika
- ¼ teaspoon crushed red pepper (dried)
- 12 sage leaves (must be fresh)

Method:
1. In a small bowl, mix together the yogurt and garlic. Season with salt if required, though this is optional.
2. Divide this mixture between four plates, spreading it to coat the middle of the plate.
3. Heat the oil or butter in a small saucepan and cook the paprika, red pepper and sage for around a minute or two before removing from the heat.
4. Bring a large skillet or pan or water to a simmer and add the vinegar, returning it back to a simmer afterwards.
5. Crack the eggs into the water and cook for about 3 minutes until the eggs are softly cooked.
6. Using a slotted spoon, remove the eggs from the water and drain for a moment.
7. Place 2 eggs on each plate on the yogurt mixture and spoon the herbs over the top.
8. Serve immediately with pita bread.

Greek Omelette

This is another filling breakfast that is packed full of the beneficial ingredients of the Mediterranean Diet. This recipe will serve 4 people and will take around 20 minutes to make. If you prefer your onions less well cooked then add them towards the end of the cooking process at the same time as the olives.

Ingredients:
- 10 eggs
- 3½oz feta cheese (crumbled)
- 3 tomatoes (coarsely chopped)
- 1 purple onion (cut into wedges)
- ½ cup fresh parsley (chopped)
- ¼ cup pitted black olives
- 2 tablespoons extra virgin olive oil

Method:
1. Preheat your grill or broiler to a high heat.
2. Whisk the eggs and parsley together in a large bowl and season with pepper and salt (the latter is optional).
3. Heat the oil in a non-stick frying pan and cook the onion wedges on a high heat for around 4 minutes until they begin to brown at the edges.
4. Add the olives and tomatoes and cook for a further 2 minutes until the tomatoes soften.
5. Reduce the heat to a medium level and then add the eggs.
6. Stir the eggs as they begin to set for about 2 minutes until half cooked, i.e. still runny in places.
7. Scatter the feta cheese over the egg and then put the pan under the grill for around 5 minutes until it puffs up and turns a golden color.
8. Serve immediately from the pan cut in to wedges.

Low Fat Mediterranean Omelette

This is another variation on the omelette which incorporates many Mediterranean vegetables for a hearty but healthy breakfast. This recipe serves 2 people and will take around 15 minutes to prepare. You can add or remove vegetables as you like.

Ingredients:

- 3 mushrooms (sliced)
- 2 eggs
- 2 marinated artichoke hearts (sliced)
- 1 asparagus stalk (soft parts sliced)
- ½ green bell pepper (diced)
- ¾ cup egg white
- ½ cup parmesan cheese (shredded)
- 1 tablespoon extra-virgin olive oil (divided)
- ½ tablespoon milk
- ¼ teaspoon balsamic vinegar

Method:
1. Whisk the eggs and milk together in a bowl and put to one side.
2. Heat the oil in a small skillet and sauté the vegetables in half the olive oil and balsamic vinegar for 4 or 5 minutes until softened and then put to one side.
3. Coat another pan with the rest of the olive oil and heat.
4. Once it has heated, pour the egg mixture in.
5. When the surface looks firm, put the vegetables and cheese on one half of the omelette and then fold the other half over it.
6. Cook for another two minutes and serve immediately.

Breakfast Casserole

This is another variation on the breakfast casserole that uses pork rather than beef, but you can reduce the pork content and add bacon if you prefer that flavor. This is a big family breakfast and will serve 10 people and takes a total of 2½ hours to cook, but is a great, filling breakfast for a weekend or when you have guests. It will also store for three days in your refrigerator so can be used for more than one breakfast.

Ingredients:

- 8 large eggs
- 8 slices wholemeal bread
- 1½lb pork sausage
- 10oz can cream of mushroom soup
- 4oz can sliced mushrooms
- ½ green bell pepper (diced)
- ½ red bell pepper (diced)
- 2½ cups milk
- 2 cups cheddar cheese (grated)
- ¼ cup black olives (chopped)
- ¾ teaspoon mustard powder

Method:
1. Remove the crust from the bread and cut into 2" cubes.
2. Spray a 9x13" casserole dish with oil and put the bread cubes in to the bottom of it.
3. Brown the sausages under a grill and slice in to a pan.
4. Add the olives and chopped peppers and heat through.
5. In a separate bowl, beat together the eggs, 2 cups of milk and the dry mustard.
6. Build layers in the casserole dish of the sausage mixture followed by cheese, followed by mushrooms, repeating until the ingredients are used up.
7. Pour the egg mixture over the dish, cover and refrigerate overnight.
8. In another bowl mix the soup and final ½ cup of milk and pour over the dish just before baking.
9. Preheat your oven to 350F and back for between 1½ and 2 hours until the egg mixture is thoroughly cooked.

Breakfast Quiche

This is very different take on breakfast and is nice on a lazy Sunday morning. It will serve 6, making it ideal for when you have guests and takes about 90 minutes to make.

Ingredients:
- 3 large eggs
- 1 zucchini (chopped)
- ¼lb mushrooms (cleaned and sliced)
- 4ozs sun dried tomatoes (drained and chopped)
- 3oz feta cheese (crumbled)
- 1 cup yellow onion (sliced)
- 1¼ cups of half and half
- ½ cup Gruyere cheese (grated)
- 3 tablespoons fresh basil (chopped)
- 2 tablespoons unsalted butter
- 2 teaspoons fresh thyme (chopped)
- 1 teaspoon garlic (minced)
- ½ teaspoon crushed red pepper
- ½ teaspoon salt
- ¼ teaspoon black pepper

Pie Crust Ingredients:
- 8oz flour
- 4oz butter (cold and cut into ¼" pieces)
- 3 tablespoons ice water
- 2 tablespoons solid vegetable shortening
- ½ teaspoon salt

Pie Crust Method:
1. Sift the salt and flour into a mixing bowl and work in the butter and shortening by hand. Use your fingertips to rub the flour and fat together until it starts to form small pea sized lumps.
2. Work the ice water in to your dough carefully and try not to mix too much until it comes together into a big lump.
3. Remove the dough (flour your hands to prevent it sticking) from the bowl and wrap in plastic wrap. Refrigerate for a minimum of 30 minutes.
4. Turn out on to a floured surface and roll into an 11" circle.
5. Put this in a 9" pie pan and trim the excess, crimping the edges in order to fit the pan.
6. Cover the bottom with parchment paper and use either pie weights or uncooked beans and cook at 350F for around 12 minutes.
7. Remove from the oven and remove the paper and weights and allow to cook for a few minutes before filling.

Quiche Method:
1. Preheat your oven to 375F.
2. Melt the butter in a large skillet and sauté the onions and zucchini for around 6 minutes.
3. Add the mushrooms and cook for another 10 minutes until the liquid is rendered.
4. Add the garlic and cook for another minute.
5. Add the basil, thyme and tomatoes and cook, stirring often, for another minutes, seasoning to taste with salt and pepper. Remove from the heat and allow to cool.
6. In a separate bowl beat the half and half with the eggs, adding the salt, pepper, crushed red pepper and Gruyere cheese.
7. Put the vegetable mixture in to the piecrust and then pour in the egg mixture.
8. Top with the crumbled goats cheese and bake until set (25-30 minutes).
9. Remove from the oven and cool for 30 minutes before serving.

MEDITERRANEAN LUNCH RECIPES

Lunch in the Mediterranean is a relaxed affair, often involving a café, friends and some socialization. In the West this may not be possible due to work commitments and the sheer chaotic nature of many of our lives.

However busy your day is, that does not stop you from having a delicious lunch that is healthy and will promote your wellbeing. There are a variety of different lunches here, many of which can be brought to an office and either eaten cold or heated up. Just because you work all day does not mean you have to go without a healthy lunch!

Some of these recipes, such as the soups, may be made in large quantities and then frozen in portion sized containers. These can be taken out of the freezer and heated up for a quick and easy healthy lunch!

Lentil Soup

Lentil soup is a delicious and quick soup to prepare that is great served with wholemeal bread or even pita bread (see later on for bread recipes).

Ingredients:
- 5 cups water
- 1 cup red lentils
- ½ cup onion (chopped)
- 2 tablespoons salt
- 2 tablespoons extra-virgin olive oil
- 1 teaspoon cumin
- Dash of either saffron of safflower spice

Method:
1. Boil all the ingredients except the cumin for 15 minutes on a high heat.
2. Add the cumin when the lentils start to soften.
3. Cook for another 5 minutes.
4. Serve hot with a side salad and wholemeal bread.

Tangy Orange Salad

This is an interesting take on the salad with the tang of the oranges offsetting the onion and olives. This can be taken to work as a lunch; just do not put the dressing on until you are ready to eat it.

Ingredients:

- 2 Oranges, segmented
- Large handful of shredded lettuce
- ½ onion (thinly sliced – use more if you prefer)
- ½ cup black olives (sliced)
- 2 tablespoons olive oil
- 2 teaspoons lemon juice

Method:

1. Cover the bottom of a plate with lettuce and layer the oranges on top together with the onions and olives.
2. Mix the olive oil and lemon juice together as a dressing

Tomato Penne Pasta

Penne pasta makes a delicious lunch and this can be served warm or eaten cold as a pasta salad.

Ingredients:

- 12oz penne pasta
- 8 ripe tomatoes (halved, seeded and chopped)
- 1 cup chopped green onions
- Feta cheese to taste (crumbled)
- ¼ cup extra-virgin olive oil
- 1 teaspoon parsley (chopped)
- 1 teaspoon dill (chopped)

Method:

1. Mix all the ingredients except the pasta in a bowl and put to one side.
2. Boil the pasta until tender but firm.
3. Allow the pasta to cool slightly and then mix in with the rest of the ingredients.
4. Serve warm or cold.

Simple Greek Salad

This is a very quick dish to prepare and makes for a nice lunch. Feel free to add other salad ingredients including sun-dried tomatoes, roasted red peppers and other olives to make it more interesting.

Ingredients:
- 1 cup spinach (chopped)
- 1 tomato (seeded and diced)
- 2 black olives (finely chopped)
- 2 tablespoons extra-virgin olive oil
- 1 tablespoon feta cheese (crumbled)
- 1 teaspoon oregano
- ½ teaspoon lemon juice

Method:
1. Mix the olives, spinach and tomato in a bowl and sprinkle the feta cheese over the top.
2. In a small bowl mix the oil, lemon juice and oregano.
3. Drizzle the dressing on the salad when ready to serve.

Grilled Pork Sandwiches

This is a dish inspired by the Italian porchetta sandwich, with a delicious fennel flavor. This meal comes together very quickly with grilled pork tenderloin and makes enough for four people.

Ingredients:
- 1¼lb pork tenderloin (remove skin, trim fat and cut in half crosswise)
- 4 sandwich rolls (split and toasted)
- ½ cup cucumber (thinly sliced)
- ½ cup fresh dill sprigs
- 1/3 cup mayonnaise
- 3 tablespoons fennel seeds (coarsely crushed)
- 1 tablespoon extra-virgin olive oil
- ¼ teaspoon ground allspice

Method:
1. Preheat your oven to 375F.
2. In a small bowl mix half of the allspice together with half the fennel seeds. Season to taste with salt and pepper if required.
3. Stir the oil in to this mixture and then press it in to the pork.
4. Grill the pork, turning regularly until browned on all sides and 140F to 145F in the middle, which will take 17 to 21 minutes.
5. Remove the pork from the heat and place on a cutting board to rest for 5 minutes.
6. In a separate bowl mix the mayonnaise with the rest of the fennel seeds and allspice. Season with salt and pepper if required.
7. Spread the mayonnaise mixture on the rolls.
8. Thinly slice the pork crosswise and arrange on the rolls with the dill and cucumbers.

Lemon Hummus Sandwich

This is a good lunch for work and has an interesting taste, being full of flavor. This recipe will make enough for eight sandwiches so feel free to store what is left over or use it as a dip for crudités or crackers. The hummus will store for 4 days in a refrigerator in an air tight container.

Hummus Ingredients:
- 2 garlic cloves (smashed)
- 2 x 15oz cans chickpeas (drained and rinsed)
- ¼ cup lemon juice (freshly squeezed)
- 6 tablespoons extra-virgin olive oil
- 2 tablespoons tahini paste
- ¾ teaspoon salt
- ½ teaspoon ground cumin
- ¼ teaspoon black pepper

Sandwich Ingredients:
- 8 slices whole meal bread
- 1 cucumber (sliced thinly crosswise)
- 2 tomatoes (thinly slice – vine ripened have the most flavor)
- 2 carrots (peels and shredded)
- ¼ red onion (thinly sliced)
- 4 cups lettuce or greens
- 1½ cups alfalfa sprouts (loosely packed)

Method:
1. Put ¾ cup of chickpeas to one side.
2. Put the rest of the chickpeas, the olive oil, tahini paste, lemon juice, cumin and garlic in to your food blender. Season to taste with salt and pepper if required.
3. Puree until smooth, stopping regularly to scrape down the sides of the bowl.
4. Transfer the hummus to a separate bowl and gently mix in the reserved chickpeas.
5. Spread each slice of break with the hummus mixture, using around ¼ cup for each slice.
6. Top four slices with the greens (evenly divided) and then top with cucumber, tomatoes and finally the alfalfa sprouts, carrot and onion.
7. Close each sandwich using a second hummus covered slice of bread, cut in half and serve.

Fattoush (Bread Salad)

This is a dish from the Middle East and is an excellent meal during the summertime as there is no cooking involved and the flavors are bold yet fresh. You can find lavash in many supermarkets though you can substitute it with pita bread though split it before you toast it. This will make enough for 4 people and can be served as a lunch or as a side to a dinner.

Ingredients:
- 5oz Lavash
- 15oz can chickpeas (drained and rinsed)
- 8oz cherry tomatoes (halved)
- 6oz sugar snap peas (trimmed and quartered with a diagonal cut)
- 6oz feta cheese (crumbled)
- 3oz baby arugula
- 1 shallot (minced)
- ¼ cup lemon juice (fresh)
- 1/3 cup fresh mint (finely chopped)
- 7 tablespoons extra-virgin olive oil
- 2 tablespoons Peppadew peppers (minced – optional)
- ½ teaspoon granulated sugar

Method:
1. Place a rack in the middle of your oven and preheat it to 350F.
2. Bake the lavash for 5 to 7 minutes until lightly browned. Remove it from the heap and allow it to crisp.
3. In the meantime, whisk the sugar, shallot and lemon juice in a bowl with a twist of pepper and pinch of salt. Leave it to sit for 10 minutes before whisking in the mint and olive oil.
4. In a large bowl mix the peas, tomatoes and chickpeas and toss with the vinaigrette from the previous step.
5. Crumble the lavash coarsely over the top.
6. Add the feta, peppers and arugula, toss to ensure thoroughly combined and server immediately.

Chickpea And Feta Za'atar Salad

Za'atar is a spice from the Middle East which has a delectable thyme and oregano flavor, making this salad a tasty, herbal treat. You can garnish this salad with red onion and / or Kalamata olives if you wish. If you want the meal to have something a little bit more special, add a tablespoon of chopped mint and some lemon zest. This recipe will make enough to serve 6 people.

Ingredients:

- 15oz can chickpeas (drained, rinsed and dried)
- 1lb cherry tomatoes (halved)
- 3oz feta cheese (crumbled)
- 3 tablespoons extra-virgin olive oil
- 1 tablespoon white wine vinegar
- 2 teaspoon za'atar
- Pinch of crushed red pepper flakes

Method:
1. In a small bowl mix together a tablespoon of the oil with the feta cheese, za'atar and red pepper flakes. Leave it to one side to site whilst you prepare the rest of the salad.
2. In a large bowl mix the tomatoes and chickpeas, seasoning with ¼ teaspoon of salt and a few twists of black pepper.
3. Add the rest of the oil and the vinegar to this mixture and then stir in the feta cheese mixture before serving.

Chickpea Burgers

This is a really nice meal that is very good for you with the combination of chickpeas, garlic, lemon and tahini sure to make you turn your back on beef burgers! These are a great lunch and this recipe will make 6 burgers. It goes well with a side salad. You may want to leave the burgers in the fridge for a half hour before cooking so they set fully as sometimes they can be a little sticky.

Ingredients:

- 1 egg
- 4 garlic cloves (sliced)
- 4 whole meal pita breads
- 2 x 15oz cans chickpeas (drained and rinsed)
- 1 tomato (thinly sliced)
- ¼ English cucumber (thinly sliced)
- ¼ cup lemon juice (fresh is best)
- ¼ cup extra-virgin olive oil (plus more to brush)
- 5 tablespoons tahini
- 2 tablespoons fresh cilantro (chopped)
- 2 tablespoons flat leaf parsley (chopped)
- 2 teaspoons ground cumin
- Harissa or other hot sauce (optional)

Method:
1. Preheat your grill or prepare your gas grill barbecue to cook these.
2. In a small saucepan heat the oil and sauté the cumin and garlic until the garlic starts to soften (around 3 minutes). Put to one side off the heat.
3. Toast one of the pita breads (under the grill or in a toaster) until crisp and golden brown. Grind to breadcrumbs in a food processor and measure; you need ½ a cup.
4. In your food processor puree a can of chickpeas with the oil mixture and 2 tablespoons of tahini, 1 tablespoon of lemon juice and the egg, adding about ¾ of a teaspoon of salt. Puree until smooth.
5. Add the rest of the chickpeas, parsley, cilantro and the pita crumbs to the food processor. Pulse until well blended and coarsely chopped.
6. In a small bowl, whisk together 2 tablespoons of water, 3 tablespoons of lemon juice and 3 tablespoons of tahini until it becomes smooth.
7. Shape the chickpea mixture into patties – it should make 6 around ¾" thick.
8. Brush both sides of the burgers with oil and grill for 2 to 3 minutes on both sides.
9. Slice 3 pita breads in half and heat briefly.
10. Place the burgers in the pita and layer with cucumber and tomatoes and drizzle with the tahini sauce and harissa before serving immediately.

Greek Salad Pita Breads

This is a great sandwich for taking on a picnic or to work for lunch. It's very easy to make and just ensure the salad is stored separately until you are ready to eat the pitas; it just stops it from getting soggy. This recipe will make enough for four people and goes very well with zucchini fritters (the next recipe).

Tapenade Ingredients:
- 1 garlic clove
- ½ cup Kalamata olives (pitted)
- 1 tablespoons extra-virgin olive oil
- 1½ teaspoons red wine vinegar.

Sandwich Ingredients:
- 4 cups spinach leaves (lightly packed)
- 1½ cups English cucumber (seeded and finely diced)
- 1¼ cups Roma tomatoes (seeded and finely diced)
- ¾ cup feta cheese (crumbled)
- ½ cup radishes (finely diced)
- 4 whole wheat pita bread (warmed)
- 2 tablespoons extra-virgin olive oil
- 1 tablespoon red wine vinegar
- 1 teaspoon dried oregano

Method:
1. For the tapenade, put the garlic in a food processor and blend until chopped. Then add the rest of the tapenade ingredients and process until they are chunky and spreadable.
2. In a large bowl mix together the tomatoes, cucumber, feta cheese and radishes.
3. Add the oregano, vinegar and olive oil, seasoning to taste with freshly ground black pepper. Toss well to combine.
4. Slice the pitas to open the pockets.
5. Divide the tapenade mixture evenly between the pitas, spreading it around the inside.
6. Put ½ cup each of the salad and spinach into each pitta and serve.

Zucchini Fritters

These are a great addition to a meal and can be served warm or cold (without the cheeses). For some variety you can add in corn for a sweeter taste. This recipe will make between 14 and 18 fritters depending on how you size them. Whilst frying the fritters, keep the ones you have already made warm in the oven until they are all ready to be served.

Ingredients:
- 1lb zucchini (coarsely grated)
- 1 cup yellow onion (finely chopped)
- 1 cup olive oil (for frying)
- ½ cup all-purpose flour
- ¼ cup fennel stalks and leaves (finely chopped)
- ¼ cup feta cheese (crumbled)
- ¼ cup Parmigianino Reggiano cheese (grated)
- 1 tablespoon fresh dill (chopped)
- 1 teaspoon baking powder
- ½ teaspoon fresh oregano (chopped)
- 1/8 teaspoon nutmeg (grated)

Method:
1. Grate the zucchini and squeeze out as much of the liquid as you can then leave it on kitchen towel to dry further.
2. Mix together the zucchini, flour, onion, fennel, baking powder, dill, nutmeg and oregano together with ½ teaspoon salt and a dash of pepper (to taste).
3. Mix well until it is moist enough to easily turn into patty shapes.
4. Each fritter is made from 2 good sized tablespoons of the mixture in a 3" diameter patty about ¼" thick.
5. Arrange the fritters on a cookie sheet until you are ready to fry them.
6. Heat the oil in a skillet (it needs to be about ¼" deep) until it starts to ripple.
7. Add the patties to the pan making sure they are not crowded or touching.
8. Fry, flipping once, for 2 or 3 minutes per side until golden brown.
9. Transfer the fritters to a plate with paper towels on to drain excess oil.
10. Repeat the frying (using more oil as required) until all the fritters are cooked.
11. Arrange the fritters on a plate (without paper towels), sprinkle with the cheese and serve warm.

Falafel Sandwich

These falafels are seared in a pan rather than deep fried, meaning they are healthier and less messy. They are served in a pita bread with tahini or a thick yogurt as a sauce. This recipe will make enough for 4 servings. As a variation on this recipe you can give your falafels a crunchier coating by breading them before cooking. If you prefer your falafel softer then reduce the cooking time by up to 30 seconds. Some cilantro or mint added to the mixture gives it an extra herby taste that you may enjoy!

Ingredients:

- 15oz can of chickpeas (drained and rinsed)
- 1 pickling cucumber (halved and sliced)
- 4 whole wheat pita breads (warmed)
- 1 onion (diced)
- 1¼ cups cherry tomatoes (cut into quarters)
- ½ cup dry breadcrumbs
- 7 tablespoons extra-virgin olive oil
- 1 tablespoon lemon juice (ideally fresh)
- 1 teaspoon ground cumin
- ½ teaspoon ground cilantro

Method:

1. Preheat your oven to 425F.
2. In your food processor mix together the chickpeas, 2 tablespoons of oil together with the cilantro and cumin. Season to taste with salt and pepper and pulse until it becomes a chunky paste.
3. Add the breadcrumbs and onion and continue to blend until it thickens up and can easily be formed in to a patty – you may need to add extra breadcrumbs.
4. Carefully make 12 patties out of the mixture, each one ½" thick.
5. Heat 2 tablespoons of oil in a non-stick pan until it starts to shimmer.
6. Add as many patties as the pan will take without crowding.
7. Cook for 2 minutes before flipping and cooking for another 2 minutes until both sides are browned. Then transfer to a baking sheet.
8. Repeat with more oil until all the patties have been fried.
9. Place all the patties on the baking sheet in the oven for 5 to 7 minutes until heated through.
10. Whilst these are cooking, toss the cucumber and tomatoes in a bowl with the lemon juice and 1 tablespoon of oil. Season with salt and pepper to taste if required.
11. Split the pita breads and stuff them with falafel and salad. Serve immediately.

Parmesan French Toast

This is a great take on firm breakfast favorite which makes for a really taste meal served with some tapenade and arugula. It makes for an ideal side or lunch and this recipe will serve 4 people.

Ingredients:
- 8 x ¾" slices of ciabatta bread
- 4 eggs
- 5oz baby arugula
- 2oz Parmigiano-Reggiano cheese (grated)
- ½ cup full fat milk
- ¼ cup tapenade (home-made or store bought)
- 1 tablespoon fresh thyme (minced)
- 1 tablespoon extra-virgin olive oil
- 1 tablespoon unsalted butter (softened)
- 1 tablespoon lemon juice (fresh is best)
- ¼ teaspoon honey
- ¼ teaspoon Tabasco (or similar) sauce

Method:
1. Preheat your oven to 425F and place a rack in the middle of your oven. Grease a large rimmed baking tray.
2. Mix together the eggs, milk, cheese, Tabasco and thyme, seasoning to taste (if required) with salt and pepper. Pour into a 9x13" baking dish.
3. Put the bread in to this dish, turn to ensure both sides are coated and leave to sit for a further 5 minutes, turning once half way through.
4. Arrange the bread on the greased baking sheet and sprinkle any leftover cheese over the top of it (you may want to grate more cheese to make this cheesier).
5. Bake in the oven for around 8 minutes until the bottom of the bread is golden. Flip and then bake for a further 5 minutes.
6. Whilst this is cooking get a large bowl and mix together the honey and lemon juice together with a few twists of black pepper and a dash of salt (if required). Whisk in the olive oil then add the arugula and toss until thoroughly coated.
7. Serve the toast with the salad and the tapenade as a side.

Lamb Shawarma

This is a Middle Eastern sandwich made with flatbread that is very easy to prepare ahead of time and assemble when required. Pomegranate molasses can be found at a Middle Eastern market or sometimes in larger supermarkets or health food stores. The sauce can be made a couple of days before needed and refrigerated until required, as can the cabbage and lamb. Reheat the lamb gently before use and allow the sauce and cabbage to return to room temperature before use.

These sandwiches can be served with pickles and anything like a chickpea salad, eggplant dip, tabbouleh or a fattoush for a larger meal. The recipe below will make enough for 6 portions.

Ingredients:
- 4 lamb shoulder chops (with bones in and around 10oz in weight)
- 4 cloves of garlic (smashed and peeled)
- 6 x 9" whole wheat flour tortillas (warmed)
- 1 carrot (sliced)
- 1 onion (cut into 8 wedges)
- 1½ cups water or dry white wine
- 2 tablespoons pomegranate molasses
- 2 tablespoons unsalted butter
- 1 tablespoon vegetable oil
- 1 tablespoon ground cumin
- 1½ teaspoons fresh lemon juice

Tahini Sauce Ingredients:
- 2 cloves of garlic (minced)
- ½ cup tahini
- ½ cup Greek yogurt (full fat)
- 3 tablespoons extra-virgin olive oil
- 2 tablespoons lemon juice (fresh)

Pickled Cabbage Ingredients:
- 2 cups red cabbage (thinly sliced)
- 1 tablespoon sherry vinegar
- ½ teaspoon pomegranate molasses
- ¼ teaspoon granulated sugar

Method:

Baising The Lamb
1. Place a rack in the middle of your oven and pre-heat to 350F.
2. Pat the lamb chops dry with paper towels.
3. Heat the vegetable oil in a large skillet and cook the lamb chops (in two batches) for about 4 minutes on each side, using more oil if required.
4. Season with salt and pepper (if required) and transfer to a 9x13" roasting dish.
5. Add a cup of wine (or water) to the skillet and simmer, scraping the pan to loosen any browned bits. Pour this wine over the chops.
6. Sprinkle the cumin over the chops followed by the carrot, onion, garlic and remaining wine (or water) so that the liquid comes about halfway up the chops. If it does not, add more water until it does.
7. Cover the pan with aluminum foil and cook for between 1½ and 2 hours until it the meat is tender.

Tahini Sauce:
1. In a medium bowl mix the lemon juice and garlic and leave to "stew" for 5 minutes.
2. Whisk in the olive oil, tahini and yogurt, adding some salt if required. Add a tablespoon or two of water (if required) to make the tahini thick but pourable.

Pickled Cabbage:
1. Heat the oil in a skillet and cook the cabbage for about 10 minutes, stirring occasionally, until it is tender.
2. Remove from the heat and stir in with the rest ingredients, seasoning to taste.

Main Dish:
1. Remove the lamb chops from the pan and cover them with aluminum foil to keep them warm.
2. Strain the roasting pan contents through a sieve into a bowl so you have around 2 cups of liquid. Discard the solid material.
3. Put the liquid in the freezer for around 15 minutes until the fat rises to the surface. Skim the fat off and discard it.
4. Boil the liquid for 10 minutes in a saucepan until it is reduced by half.
5. Break the lamb into small chunks (you can use your fingers) and get rid of the fat and bones.
6. In a separate bowl whisk together the butter, braising juices, lemon juice and pomegranate molasses.
7. Add the lamb and mix well to ensure thoroughly coated. Season to taste with salt and pepper if required.
8. Divide the lamb evenly between the tortillas.
9. Top the lamb with 2 or 3 tablespoons (to taste) of sauce and cabbage before rolling it up firmly like a burrito wrap. Rest it on its seam side to keep it closed whilst you repeat this with the rest.
10. Heat a non-stick pan and cook the shawarma with the seam side down until brown and crisp (about 3 minutes). Do not flip them over.
11. Serve immediately.

Spicy Lamb Burgers

This is a delicious meal, flavored with warm spices offset by the salad and yogurt. It will serve 4 people and if you do not like lamb then feel free to substitute with ground beef instead. For a fuller flavor you can mix the topping paste with Greek Yogurt and even add some crumbled feta cheese.

Ingredients:
- 1½lbs ground lamb (beef can be substituted)
- 1 garlic clove (minced)
- 2 x 6" whole wheat pita breads (halved and warmed)
- ¼ cup fresh cilantro (packed)
- ¼ cup flat leaf parsley (packed)
- 2 tablespoons fresh oregano (packed)
- 1 tablespoon sherry vinegar
- 1 tablespoon plus ¼ cup extra-virgin olive oil (more required for the grill)
- 1 teaspoon each of ginger, ground cumin and ground coriander
- ½ teaspoon crushed red pepper flakes
- ½ teaspoon ground cinnamon
- Plain Greek yogurt (for serving)
- Sliced tomato (for serving)

Method:
1. Prepare a gas or charcoal grill to a medium high heat.
2. In a large bowl mix the lamb together with a tablespoon of olive oil, cinnamon, ginger, cumin and coriander. Season to taste with salt and pepper and mix thoroughly.
3. Form into 4 patties, each ½" thick.
4. Oil your grill grate and grill each burger for 5 minutes, then flip and grill for a further 5 minutes. An instant read thermometer should have a reading of 145F after this for a medium cooked burger.
5. In a food processor mix the sherry vinegar, parsley, cilantro, oregano, garlic and red pepper flakes together with the ¼ cup of olive oil, seasoning to taste.
6. Pulse until it forms a coarse paste and scrape the sides of the processor to ensure it is well mixed.
7. Each burger is served in half a pita with sauce, tomato and Greek Yogurt.

Fried Egg Pitas

This is a Mediterranean version of the fried egg sandwich with a twist from the salty olive and caper tapenade. You can make your own or you can buy it pre-made from a supermarket (usually found near the olives). This recipe will make 4 sandwiches, plenty for a good lunch or even an alternative breakfast!

Ingredients:
- 2 whole wheat pita (halved and warmed)
- 4 eggs
- 1 cup baby arugula (lightly packed)
- ¼ cup tapenade
- 2 tablespoons extra-virgin olive oil

Method:
1. Heat the oil in a non-stick pan.
2. Once it has heated, break the eggs in to the pan and cook to your preference (3 or 4 minutes for sunny side up or flip and cook for another minute for over easy).
3. Whilst the eggs are cooking, open the pitas and spread the tapenade on the inside and divide the arugula between the pitas.
4. Sprinkle the cooked eggs with salt and pepper (if required) and transfer to the pita.

Fennel And Tomato Soup

This is a nice variation of the perennial favorite, tomato soup. The fennel provides a delicious aniseed flavor that offsets the sweetness of the tomato nicely. If you prefer you can use peeled and de-seeded fresh tomatoes instead of canned. This will make enough soup for 4 servings and will work well served with a whole wheat rustic bread. This can be made even more delicious by mashing some goats cheese, mixing it with some chopped fresh parsley, spreading it on the bread and then toasting the bread in a broiler for a few minutes to warm the cheese. For a vegetarian version substitute vegetable stock for the chicken broth.

Ingredients:
- 28oz can crushed tomatoes
- 1 onion (finely diced)
- 1 cup canned chicken broth
- ½ cup low fat milk
- ¼ cup orange juice (fresh)
- 2 tablespoons unsalted butter
- ½ teaspoon whole fennel seeds (chopped)
- Pinch of crushed red pepper flakes

Method:
1. Melt the butter in a large saucepan over a medium heat.
2. Add the onions and cook until soft but not brown (around 5 minutes), stirring often.
3. Add the fennel seeds and red pepper flakes and cook for another 1 minutes.
4. Add the chicken broth, tomatoes and orange juice.
5. Bring the pan to a boil and then reduce the heat and simmer for a further 15 minutes.
6. Remove the soup from the heat and use a hand blender to blend it in the pan or blend it in your food processor.
7. Blend until smooth and add the milk. If the soup is too thick add more chicken broth to thin it out.
8. If necessary, reheat prior to serving.

MEDITERRANEAN DINNER RECIPES

Dinner in the Mediterranean is typically a leisurely and social affair, often accompanied by a glass or two of red wine. The red wine (or red grape juice) is an essential part of the Mediterranean diet as it is jam packed with anti-oxidants that are vital for your health.

This chapter will introduce you to some of the main courses that you can make, many of which can be served with rustic bread, olives, side salads, roasted Mediterranean vegetables and some of the ideas from earlier in this book.

Chicken Pasta – Grecian Style

This is a great variation on the pasta dish which incorporates the flavors of Greece, making for a very satisfying meal. You can add some Kalamata olives which will give it some extra flavor and use any type of pasta. This recipe will make enough for 6 servings.

Ingredients:

- 16oz pasta (any variety)
- 1lb chicken breast (diced – skin and bones removed)
- 14oz can marinated artichoke hearts (drained and chopped)
- 2 garlic cloves (crushed)
- 1 tomato (chopped)
- ½ cup red onion (chopped)
- ½ cup feta cheese (crumbled)
- 3 tablespoons fresh parsley (chopped)
- 2 tablespoons lemon juice
- 1 tablespoon olive oil
- 2 teaspoons dried oregano
- 2 lemon wedges (for serving)

Method:
1. Boil a pan of water and cook the pasta for between 8 and 10 minutes until it is tender but firm, then drain it.
2. Heat the oil in a non-stick pan over a medium to high heat and sauté the onion and garlic for 2 minutes until fragrant.
3. Add the chicken and cook for around 6 minutes, stirring occasionally, until the juices run clear and the chicken is not pink in the middle.
4. Reduce the heat to a lower setting and add the pasta (cooked), artichoke hearts, feta cheese, tomato, lemon juice, parsley and oregano.
5. Stir well and cook for another 3 minutes until heated through.
6. Serve immediately garnished with lemon wedges.

Spinach Pita Bake

This can be a full meal served with salad, couscous or similar side dish and makes a good appetizer as well. It is full of flavor and has a delicious crunch crush. You can add or remove vegetables as you see fit and even change the cheese if you prefer. This meal will make enough for 6 servings.

Ingredients:
- 6 whole wheat pita breads
- 6ox tub sun-dried tomato pesto
- 4 mushrooms (sliced)
- 2 plum (Roma) tomatoes (chopped)
- 1 bunch spinach (rinsed and roughly chopped)
- ½ cup feta cheese (crumbled)
- 3 tablespoons olive oil
- 2 tablespoons Parmesan cheese (grated)

Method:
1. Preheat your oven to 350F.
2. Spread one side of each pita with tomato pesto and place them on a baking sheet with the pesto side up.
3. Top each pita with some spinach, tomato, mushroom and cheese then drizzle with olive oil. Season to taste with freshly ground black pepper.
4. Bake for around 12 minutes until the pita breads are crisp, remove from the oven and cut in to quarters.

Greek Potatoes

This is a simple recipe that comes out of Greece. You can adjust this recipe to your own tastes, adding a little bit more lemon if you like. These potatoes are great when served with green beans or roasted chicken breasts with salsa and crumbled feta cheese. The recipe will make enough for 4 servings. If you want to make the potatoes a little drier then remove the foil about 10 or 15 minutes before the potatoes are cooked.

Ingredients:
- 6 potatoes (peeled and quartered)
- 2 cubes chicken bouillon (vegetable stock can be used instead)
- 2 garlic cloves (finely chopped)
- Juice of 1 lemon
- 1½ cups water
- 1/3 cup olive oil
- 1 teaspoon dried rosemary
- 1 teaspoon dried thyme or oregano

Method:
1. Preheat your oven to 350F.
2. In a small bowl mix together the water, olive oil, lemon juice, garlic, thyme, rosemary and bouillon cubes. Season to taste with freshly ground black pepper.
3. Arrange the tomatoes on the bottom of a baking dish and pour the sauce over the top of them.
4. Turn the potatoes so they are coated in the mixture and then cover the dish with foil.
5. Cook in the oven for between 1½ and 2 hours, turning occasionally.

White Bean Pasta

This dish is full of flavors that work well together. For a bit of an extra kick add some basil, oregano, crushed red pepper flakes or garlic.

Ingredients:
- 2 x 14½oz can diced tomatoes
- 19oz can cannellini beans (drained and rinsed)
- 10oz fresh spinach (washed and roughly chopped)
- 8oz penne pasta (or other variety)
- ½ cup feta cheese (crumbled)

Method:
1. Cook the pasta in a large pan of boiling water for 8 to 10 minutes, then drain and put to one side.
2. Boil the beans and tomatoes in a large non-stick pan then reduce the heat and simmer for 10 minutes.
3. Add the spinach and cook for a further 2 minutes until the spinach wilts, stirring constantly.
4. Divide the pasta between three or four plates, pour the source over the top and sprinkle with the feta cheese.

Pasta Fagioli

This is a traditional Italian soup that makes for a delicious meal! It is best served with some garlic bread and a mixed leaf salad to turn it in to a full meal but can be used on its own as a lunch or a starter. Serve garnished with grated Parmesan cheese. This recipe will make enough for 4 servings.

Ingredients:
- 15oz can cannellini beans (keep the liquid)
- 14½oz can chicken broth
- 8oz can tomato sauce (or home-made sauce can be used)
- 3 garlic cloves (minced)
- 2 celery stalks (chopped)
- 2 tomatoes (peeled and chopped)
- 1 onion (chopped)
- 1/2 cup spinach pasta (uncooked)
- 1 tablespoon olive oil
- 2 teaspoons dried parsley
- 1 teaspoon Italian seasoning
- ¼ teaspoon crushed red pepper flakes

Method:
1. Heat the oil in a large saucepan and sauté the garlic, onion, celery, parsley, red pepper flakes and Italian seasoning for around 5 minutes until the onion turns translucent.
2. Add the tomatoes, tomato sauce and chicken broth and simmer for another 15 to 20 minutes.
3. Add the pasta and cook for a further 10 minutes until it becomes tender.
4. Add the beans and the liquid and mix thoroughly. Cook until heated through and serve immediately.

Tasty Greek Salad

This is a very tasty and healthy salad that makes a great accompaniment to any of the meals in this book. It can also be used as a lunch with some roast chicken breast to bulk it out. You can stir in a couple of tablespoons of low fat Greek yogurt to make the salad creamier. This recipe makes enough for 6 servings.

Ingredients:
- 6 Kalamata olives (pitted and sliced)
- 3 large tomatoes (chopped)
- 2 cucumbers (peeled and chopped)
- 1 red onion (chopped – substitute for 2 green onions if preferred)
- ½ green pepper (chopped)
- 1 cup feta cheese (crumbled)
- ¼ cup olive oil
- 3 teaspoons lemon juice
- 1½ teaspoons dried oregano
- 1 teaspoon red wine vinegar
- ¼ teaspoon each of salt and pepper

Method:
1. Mix the onion, cucumber and tomatoes in a salad bowl and stir until well combined.
2. Add the rest of the ingredients and stir well before serving.

Mediterranean Chicken

This is a delicious dish where the chicken is full of flavor. The recipe will make enough for 6 servings. For some extra flavor you can add artichoke hearts and some feta cheese or even some crushed red pepper flakes to spice it up a little. If you prefer you can slice the chicken in to strips rather than have the breast halves, though adjust any cooking times accordingly.

Ingredients:
- 6 chicken breast halves (skin and bone removed)
- 3 garlic cloves (minced)
- 3 cups tomatoes (chopped)
- ½ cup onion (diced)
- ½ cup white wine
- ½ cup Kalamata olives (chopped)
- ¼ cup fresh parsley (chopped)
- 2 tablespoons white wine
- 1 tablespoon fresh basil (chopped)
- 2 teaspoons fresh thyme (chopped)
- 2 teaspoons olive oil

Method:
1. Heat the oil and 2 tablespoons of white wine in a large pan over a medium heat.
2. Add the chicken and cook for about 5 minutes on each side until golden then remove the chicken from the heat and put to one side.
3. Cook the garlic in the same pan using the chicken juices for half a minute before adding the onion and cooking for another 3 minutes.
4. Add the tomatoes and then bring the pan to the boil.
5. Reduce the heat and add the ½ cup of white wine and simmer for another 10 minutes.
6. Add the basil and thyme and simmer for a further 5 minutes.
7. Add the chicken to the pan and cover, cooking for another 10-15 minutes until the chicken is thoroughly cooked and not pink on the inside.
8. Add the olives and parsley and cook for a further minute.
9. Serve immediately and season to taste with salt and pepper if required.

Shrimp Pasta

This is a lovely dish that incorporates seafood in to your diet. It is an interesting pasta dish and is a nice change from the usual pasta dishes people eat. This recipe will make enough for 8 people.

Ingredients:
- 16oz penne pasta (use an alternative if you prefer)
- 2 x 14oz cans diced tomatoes
- 1lb shrimp (peeled and deveined)
- 1 cup Parmesan cheese (grated)
- ¼ cup red onion (chopped)
- ¼ cup white wine
- 2 tablespoons olive oil
- 1 tablespoon chopped garlic
- ½ teaspoon each of red pepper flakes, garlic powder and parsley (optional)

Method:
1. Add the pasta to a pan of boiling water and cook for between 8 and 10 minutes until al dente then drain.
2. Heat the oil in a pan over a medium heat and sauté the onion and garlic for 4 to 5 minutes until tender.
3. Add the tomatoes and wine and cook for a further 10 minutes, stirring occasionally.
4. Add the shrimp, stir well and cook for a further 5 minutes until it becomes opaque.
5. Toss in with the pasta and cheese then serve.

Creamy White Bean Soup

This is a hearty but healthy soup that will make enough for 4 servings. It sounds like it is difficult to make but is actually very easy to cook. It can be served garnished with some grated Parmesan cheese.

Ingredients:
- 2 x 16oz cans white kidney beans (drained and rinsed)
- 14oz can chicken broth
- 1 onion (chopped)
- 1 celery stalk (chopped)
- 1 garlic clove (minced)
- 1 bunch fresh spinach (rinsed and sliced)
- 2 cups water
- 1 tablespoon lemon juice
- 1 tablespoon olive oil
- ¼ teaspoon black pepper
- Small pinch of dried thyme

Method:
1. Heat the oil in a large saucepan and sauté the celery and onion for 6 or 7 minutes until tender.
2. Add the garlic and cook, stirring continuously, for another 30 seconds.
3. Add the beans, chicken broth, water, thyme and pepper and bring to the boil.
4. Reduce the heat and simmer for a further 15 minutes.
5. Use a slotted spoon to remove 2 cups of beans and vegetables and put to one side.
6. Use your food processor to blend the rest of the soup until smooth, in batches if required.
7. Pour this back in to the pan and add the reserved beans and vegetables.
8. Bring to the boil, stirring occasionally and add the spinach, cooking for a further minute.
9. Stir in the lemon juice and serve with grate Parmesan cheese on top.

Mediterranean Flounder

Fish features heavily in the Mediterranean diet and this is a very tasty fish dish using a fish common to the Mediterranean area but perhaps less used elsewhere. This dish is best served with green vegetables and white rice which complement the taste very well. This recipe makes enough to serve 4 people.

Ingredients:
- 5 plum tomatoes
- 2 garlic cloves (chopped)
- ½ onion (chopped)
- 24 Kalamata olives (pitted and chopped)
- 12 leaves fresh basil (6 chopped, 6 torn)
- 1lb flounder fillets
- ¼ cup capers
- ¼ cup white wine
- 3 tablespoons Parmesan cheese (grated)
- 2 tablespoons extra-virgin olive oil
- 1 teaspoon fresh lemon juice
- Pinch of Italian seasoning

Method:
1. Preheat your oven to 425F.
2. Boil a pan of water and plunge the tomatoes in to it then remove immediately to a bowl of ice water. Drain the water off and then remove the skins from the tomatoes. Discard the skins, chop the tomatoes and put to one side.
3. Heat the oil in a pan on a medium heat and sauté the onion for about 5 minutes until tender.
4. Stir in the garlic, tomatoes and the Italian seasoning. Cook for a further 5 to 7 minutes until the tomato is tender.
5. Next add the olives, capers, wine, lemon juice and half of the basil. Stir thoroughly.
6. Reduce the heat to low and blend in the parmesan cheese. Cook for around 15 minutes until the mixture reduces to a thick sauce.

7. Place the flounder in a shallow baking dish and pour the sauce over the fillets. Sprinkle the remaining basil leaves over the top.
8. Bake in your oven for around 12 minutes until the fish easily flakes with a fork and serve immediately.

Sicilian Spaghetti

This is a lovely Italian dish that will make enough to serve 8 people. It is best served with a fresh, crusty Italian bread.

Ingredients:
- 1lb spaghetti
- 3 garlic cloves (crushed)
- 2oz can anchovy fillets (chopped)
- 1 cup fine bread crumbs
- 1 cup fresh parsley (chopped)
- 6 tablespoons olive oil
- 4 tablespoons Parmesan cheese (grated)

Method:
1. Boil a pan of water (lightly salted if desired) and cook the pasta for between 8 and 10 minutes until cooked. Then drain.
2. Whilst this is cooking, heat the oil in a pan over a medium heat and cook the anchovies and garlic for 2 minutes, stirring constantly.
3. Stir in the breadcrumbs then remove the mixture from the heat.
4. Mix in the parsley and season with freshly ground black pepper.
5. Toss the anchovy mixture in with the hot spaghetti, sprinkle with cheese and serve.

Spanish Cod

This is a delicious fish dish with a strong tomato sauce and some marinated vegetables. This recipe will serve 6 people. You can make the meal even more filling by using some jumbo shrimp too. The cod can be substituted for any other white fish if you prefer.

Ingredients:
- 6 x 4oz cod fillets
- 15 cherry tomatoes (halved)
- 1 cup tomato sauce
- ½ cup green olives (chopped)
- ¼ cup marinated Italian vegetable salad (from a deli is best – drain it and chop it coarsely before using)
- ¼ cup onion (finely chopped)
- 2 tablespoons garlic (chopped)
- 1 tablespoon extra-virgin olive oil
- 1 tablespoon butter
- Dash each of paprika, cayenne pepper and black pepper

Method:
1. In a large skillet heat the butter and oil on a medium heat, cooking the garlic and onions for 3 or 4 minutes until the onions are tender but the garlic is not burnt.
2. Add the cherry tomatoes and the tomato sauce and then bring the mixture to a simmer.
3. Stir in the olives, vegetables and seasonings (to taste).
4. Add the cod fillets and cook for about 8 minutes until the fish is easily flaked by a fork and then serve immediately.

Spanish Mediterranean Chicken

This dish is influenced by the cuisine of the northern Mediterranean part of Spain where the saltiness of the olives compliments the sweetness of the pineapple. This dish makes enough to serve 10 and is best served on a bed of rice.

Ingredients:
- 10 chicken breast halves (skinless and boneless)
- 20oz can pineapple chunks in juice (drained and juice reserved)
- 14oz can stewed tomatoes
- 2 garlic cloves (minced)
- 1 red bell pepper (thinly sliced)
- 1 onion (quartered)
- 2 cups black olives
- ½ cup salsa
- 2 tablespoons cornstarch
- 2 tablespoons water
- 1 tablespoon extra-virgin olive oil
- 1 teaspoon each of ground cinnamon and ground cumin

Method:
1. Heat the oil in a large frying pan and brown the chicken.
2. Mix the cinnamon and cumin together and sprinkle over the chicken before adding the garlic and onion, cooking for a further 5 minutes until the onion is soft.
3. Add the pineapple chunks, salsa, olives and tomatoes and simmer, covered, for 25 minutes.
4. Mix the cornstarch with the water and stir into the juice in the pan.
5. Add the bell pepper and simmer until the sauce starts to thicken.
6. Finally add the pineapple chunks and cook for another 2 to 4 minutes until heated through.
7. Serve hot on a bed of rice

Grecian Pasta Salad

Pasta salad is always a popular dish and there are plenty of variations. This particularly dish will make 8 servings but feel free to add or remove ingredients as you see fit or depending on what you have in the cupboards. It can make a good lunch, dinner or even a side for one of the other main courses detailed in this book.

Ingredients:
- 16oz penne pasta
- 2 tomatoes (chopped)
- 1 onion (chopped)
- 1 green bell pepper (chopped)
- 1 cucumber (coarsely chopped)
- 1 cup black olives (chopped)
- ¼ cup extra-virgin olive oil
- 1 teaspoon garlic salt
- 1 teaspoon dried basil
- 1 teaspoon ground black pepper
- 1 teaspoon lemon juice

Method:
1. Cook the pasta for 8 to 10 minutes in a large pan of boiling water until done then drain and rinse in cold water. Put to one side whilst preparing the rest of the meal.
2. Mix, in a small bowl, the oil, basil, black pepper, garlic salt and lemon juice.
3. In a larger bowl mix the pasta and the rest of the ingredients.
4. Add the dressing and toss well to ensure thoroughly coated.
5. Refrigerate for 30 minutes before serving.

Sausage Marsala

This is a great dish that is made using Italian sausages. These can be substituted for any other type of sausages you prefer or you can use vegetarian sausages to make this dish vegetarian friendly. If you like the taste of the Marsala wine then you can add a bit more to give the dish a fuller flavor or you can use a cabernet wine instead of Marsala if you struggle to get hold of it. This dish will make enough for 6 servings.

Ingredients:
- 16oz pasta (farfalle or penne pasta work well)
- 1lb Italian sausage links
- 14oz can diced tomatoes (undrained)
- 1 garlic clove (minced)
- 1 green bell pepper (sliced)
- 1 red bell pepper (sliced)
- ½ onion (sliced)
- 1/3 cup water
- 1 tablespoon Marsala wine
- A pinch each of dried oregano and black pepper

Method:
1. Boil a large pan of water and cook the pasta for between 8 to 10 minutes until al dente and then drain.
2. Place the water and sausages (whole) into a pan over a medium to high heat. Cover and cook for 7 to 8 minutes then drain off the juices and slice thinly.
3. Cook the sausages in the pan together with the garlic, peppers, Marsala wine and onions until the sausage is cooked through.
4. Add in the tomatoes, oregano and black pepper and cook for a further 2 minutes.
5. Serve immediately over the cooked pasta.

Mussels Marinara

This is a very romantic meal combining the flavors of mussels and linguine. The recipe will make enough for 4 servings and is best served with a good bottle of wine and some crusty French bread. You can make this meal more substantial by adding shrimp and scallops as well as the mussels.

Ingredients:
- 14oz can crushed tomatoes
- 1lb mussels (cleaned and de-bearded)
- 8oz linguini pasta
- 1 garlic clove (minced)
- 1 shallot (minced)
- ¼ cup white wine (red can be used if you prefer)
- 1 tablespoon extra-virgin olive oil
- ½ teaspoon each of dried oregano and dried basil
- Pinch of crushed red pepper flakes (add more for extra zing)
- 1 lemon for garnish (cut into wedges)

Method:
1. Heat the oil in a large skillet over a medium heat and sauté the shallot and garlic for 3 to 5 minutes until transparent.
2. Add the tomatoes, red pepper flakes, basil and oregano, reduce the heat to low and simmer for a further 5 minutes.
3. Whilst this is simmering, boil a large pan of water, add the pasta and cook for 8 to 10 minutes before draining and putting to one side.
4. Add the mussels and wine to the skillet, turn the heat to high and cover, cooking for 3 to 5 minutes until the shells open.
5. Divide the pasta between the plates and pour this mixture over the pasta. Sprinkle with parsley and squeeze a lemon wedge over the top.
6. Serve immediately garnished with another lemon wedge.

Roasted Vegetable Pasta

This is a delicious dish that is full of vegetables and really good for you. You can roast extra vegetables and cool the rest to use in wraps with cheese and mayo for lunch or make a bigger quantity of this dish and freeze the excess for use another day. This dish will make enough for 3 servings.

Ingredients:
- 2 red bell peppers (sliced)
- 10 garlic cloves (chopped)
- 8oz fettuccini noodles (dry)
- ½ tomato (quartered)
- ¼lb crimini mushrooms (sliced)
- ¼lb asparagus (trimmed and cut into 4" pieces)
- ¼ cup Parmesan cheese (grated)
- 2 tablespoons extra-virgin olive oil
- 2 tablespoons tapenade
- ½ teaspoon fresh oregano (chopped)
- ½ teaspoon fresh rosemary (chopped)

Method:
1. Preheat your oven to 350F.
2. Add all the vegetables to a large roasting pan and mix well.
3. Sprinkle with oregano and rosemary and then drizzle with the olive oil.
4. Bake for 15 minutes.
5. Meanwhile, boil a large pan of water and cook for the pasta for 8 to 10 minutes and then drain.
6. Mix the pasta with the roasted vegetables, tapenade and Parmesan cheese and then serve immediately.

Sicilian Lemon Chicken

This is a great dish to cook when you want to impress someone, making it ideal for a date or visitors. The sweet yet tangy sauce compliments the chicken and the garnishes give the dish a great look. One tip to help make the dish better is to flatten out the chicken breasts before frying to ensure a more even cook. For those that prefer a fuller flavor you can season the chicken breasts with salt and pepper before frying. This dish makes enough to serve 4 people.

Ingredients:
- 16oz angel hair pasta
- 15oz can diced tomatoes (drained)
- 4 chicken breast halves (skinless and boneless)
- 1 onion (halved and thinly sliced)
- Zest and juice of one lemon
- 2 bay leaves
- 4 springs fresh basil
- ¾ cup golden raisins
- ¼ Parmesan cheese shavings
- 3 tablespoons extra-virgin olive oil
- 2 tablespoons black olives (sliced)
- 2 tablespoons julienned fresh basil
- 2 tablespoons pine nuts

- 1 tablespoon balsamic vinegar
- 1 tablespoon extra-virgin olive oil
- 1 tablespoon minced garlic
- 1 teaspoon white sugar
- ¼ teaspoon cayenne pepper
- ¼ teaspoon dried oregano

Method:
1. Soak the raisins in some warm water for about 10 minutes until they fatten up. Drain and put to one side.
2. In a saucepan over a medium heat, warm 3 tablespoons of olive oil and sauté the olives, pine nuts, onion and garlic, seasoning with the oregano, cayenne pepper and bay leaves until the onions start to turn a golden color (about 5 minutes).
3. Add the tomatoes and season to taste with salt and pepper and cook for another 5 minutes, stirring occasionally.
4. Add the sugar, balsamic vinegar and raisins, cooking for another 5 minutes until thickened, stirring occasionally.
5. Carefully remove the bay leaves, add the julienned basil and stir well.
6. Cover and keep warm on a low heat.
7. Cook the pasta in a pan of boiling water for 8 to 10 minutes until cooked and then drain.
8. Meanwhile, heat the tablespoon of olive oil in a frying pan on a medium heat.
9. Whilst this is heating, toss the chicken in the lemon juice and ensure it is coated.
10. Cook the chicken for about 15 minutes in the frying pan until it is golden brown and the juice run clear.
11. Remove from the heat, transfer to a plate and rest for 5 minutes.
12. Cut the chicken breast into thin slices (against the grain works best).
13. Divide the pasta between four wide but shallow bowls and spread the chicken slices over the top in a fan shape.
14. Spoon tomato sauce over the top and sprinkle with the cheese and lemon zest. Garnish with a sprig of basil before serving.

Greek Baked Salmon

Salmon is one of the best fish you can eat, being full of Omega-3 and other vital vitamins, plus it tastes absolutely delicious! This dish is a Greek way of preparing salmon which gives it a very interesting taste. The recipe will make 8 servings.

Ingredients:
- 8 salmon fillets (5oz each, with skin)
- 4 plum tomatoes (diced)
- 4 Kalamata olives (sliced)
- ¼ red onion (diced)
- ½ cup extra-virgin olive oil
- ½ cup feta cheese (crumbled)
- ¼ cup olive oil
- 1 tablespoon lemon juice
- 1 tablespoon fresh basil (chopped)

Method:
1. Preheat your oven to 350F.
2. Brush each of the salmon fillets with olive oil, making sure they are well covered and then place in the bottom of a glass baking dish, skin side down.
3. Scatter the rest of the ingredients over the fillets and sprinkle with the lemon juice.
4. Bake for around 20 minutes in your oven until the salmon flakes easily with a fork.

Gooey Goat Cheese Figs

Don't let the title of the dish put you off because fresh figs stuffed with goats cheese is a dish made in heaven when roasted on the grill and drizzled with honey. If you want an extra special flavor then skewer each of the figs with a frond of rosemary. This recipe makes enough for 4 servings. This makes a great side for many of the dishes listed here or a delicious and very different snack to have at your next barbecue.

Ingredients:
- 8 fresh figs
- 8 grape leaves (rinsed and drained)
- ½ cup honey
- ½ cup goat cheese (softened)
- Skewers

Method:
1. Preheat your grill to a medium heat.
2. Make a small cut at the bottom of each of the figs, just large enough to hold a pastry bag tip.
3. Put the softened goat cheese in your pastry bag, using a plain tip, and fill each fig with the cheese by squeezing it in the bottom. The figs are going to plump up when they are filled.
4. Wrap a grape leaf around each fig and then put 2 or 3 figs on each skewer.
5. Lightly oil your grill grate and then cook the figs on the grill for about 3 minutes, turning once.
6. Drizzle with honey and serve immediately.

Stifado (Greek Chicken Stew)

This is a hearty Greek meal traditionally made with beef or even hare, though this version uses chicken which is lower in calories. It's a great dish to make in large quantities and freeze the rest. This recipe makes enough for 8 servings.

Shallots can easily be peeled by blanching them in boiling water until the skins loosen, which takes about 3 minutes. Then cut the ends from the shallots and take the skin off; which is much easier than fiddling around trying to peel them.

Ingredients:
- 1 chicken (4lb in weight or 4 large chicken breasts cut into bite sized pieces)
- 10 small shallots (peeled)
- 2 garlic cloves (finely chopped)
- 2 bay leaves
- 1½ cups chicken stock (more may be required)
- 1 cup tomato sauce
- 1 cup extra-virgin olive oil
- ½ cup red wine
- 2 tablespoons fresh parsley (chopped)
- 2 teaspoons butter
- Pinch of dried oregano

Method:
1. Boil the peeled shallots for 3 minutes in a pan of water until tender. Drain and plunge into ice water (or rinse with cold water for a few minutes) to stop the cooking process. Drain well and put to one side.
2. In a Dutch oven (or large pot on a medium heat) heat the oil and butter until the butter is melted and bubbling.
3. Add the whole shallots and the chicken pieces and cook for about 15 minutes until the shallots have softened and the chicken is no longer pink inside.
4. Add the garlic and cook for 3 more minutes until it starts to turn golden.
5. Add the tomato sauce, red wine, parsley, bay leaves and oregano. Season to taste with salt and pepper, if required, and stir well.
6. Pour enough chicken stock in to cover the chicken and stir well.
7. Simmer for around 50 minutes, covered, on a medium to low heat until the chicken is tender and the shallots are soft

MEDITERRANEAN DESSERT RECIPES

Dessert is considered an essential part of any meal by many of us, and it usually ends up being high calorie and very unhealthy. Mediterranean desserts are based around fresh ingredients that are a lot healthier for you, though this does not mean they are tasteless.

These desserts will do well at any dinner party and are delicious. You will enjoy the sweet tastes as well as the use of chocolate and honey to provide that taste. Many of these can be stored in your refrigerator for a few days, meaning you can easily make the desserts in advance and enjoy them for several days.

Tahini And Honey Ganache

The chocolate in this recipe is complemented surprisingly well by the toasted sesame seeds and enhanced by the use of tahini. These chocolates work well as an after dinner chocolate and complement any Egyptian or Moroccan style dish, though works with most meals. This recipe makes enough for 40 chocolates.

Ingredients:
- 12½oz of dark chocolate (at least 66% cocoa – chopped)
- ¾ cup sesame seeds
- 1/3 cup tahini
- 2½ tablespoons clover or heather honey

Method:
1. Bring ¾ cup of water and honey to a simmer in a saucepan.
2. Add the tahini and simmer for 2 more minutes.
3. Put the chocolate in to a heat proof bowl and then pour the hot liquid on to the chocolate.
4. Allow to cool and then refrigerate for 2 hours to ensure it is fully set.
5. Lightly toast the sesame seeds using a dry frying pan until they are golden but not starting to pop open. Put to one side and allow to cool.
6. Take the ganache out of the refrigerator and use a teaspoon to scoop out quenelles (don't worry about them being even).
7. Immediately roll in the toasted sesame seeds.
8. These are best served at room temperature and can be refrigerated and used within 3 days.

Raspberry And Fig Crostatas

The crostata is a popular Italian pie though the flavours are somewhat unusual, but surprisingly good! These pies can be stored for a day or two, but will be at their best when freshly made. This recipe will make 10 crostatas.

Dough Ingredients:
- 7½oz all-purpose flour (unbleached)
- 3¾oz whole wheat flour
- 9oz cold, unsalted butter (cut into small chunks)
- ¼ cup plus ½ tablespoon granulated sugar
- 1 teaspoon ground cinnamon
- ½ teaspoon salt

Filling Ingredients:
- ¾lb small fresh figs (quartered)
- 6oz fresh raspberries
- 1oz cold unsalted butter (cut into chunks)
- 1/3 cup plus 2 tablespoons granulated sugar
- 3 tablespoons plus a teaspoon of honey
- 3 tablespoons plus a teaspoon of graham cracker crumbs
- 1½ tablespoons heavy cram
- 1 tablespoon fresh thyme (chopped)
- 2 teaspoons orange zest (finely grated)

Dough Method:
1. Put both flours, salt, cinnamon and sugar in to a food processor.
2. Add the butter and pulse in short bursts until the mixture becomes a coarse meal.
3. Add 3 tablespoons of cold water and pulse again, adding more water (a tablespoon at a time) if the mixture seems dry. Pulse until the mixture comes together, though do not over-process.
4. Turn the dough out on to a clean, floured work surface and gather it together.
5. Divide the dough into ten 2½oz rounds and flatten then into disks. Wrap in plastic wrap and refrigerate for 2 hours or up to three days.
6. When ready to use preheat your oven to 400F and line two rimmed baking sheets with parchment. Place one oven shelf in the top third and a second in the bottom third.
7. On a floured surface, roll out each piece of dough into a round that is 5½ across and about 1/8 of an inch thick. Put 5 rounds on each baking sheet.

Filling Method:
1. In a large bowl toss together the raspberries, figs, honey, orange zest, thyme and 1/3 cup of sugar until well mixed.

Assembly And Baking:
1. Sprinkle a teaspoon of graham cracker crumbs at the center of each dough round leaving a border of about ½". This will soak up any excess juice and stop the pies getting soggy.
2. Put a ¼ cup of the filing mixture in the middle of each round, mounding it up and top with a slice of butter.
3. Fold the edges of the dough up and over some of the fruit to create a 1" rim which leaves the middle exposed.
4. Work your way around each dough round pleating the dough.
5. Brush the crust of each of the crostatas with cream and then sprinkle the 2 tablespoons of sugar over the crusts and filling.
6. Bake in the oven for 30 to 35 minutes, swapping and rotating the position of the baking sheets halfway through.
7. Remove the baking sheets from the oven and leave to cool for 5 minutes.
8. Using a spatula, carefully loosen the crostatas and leave to cool on the baking sheets.

Almond Tuiles

These are an exotic cookie which works well as a dessert or a snack during the day. To make this dish look fantastic, use black sesame seeds which really stand out in the cookie dough. This recipe will make 20 tuiles which are best eaten within a few hours of baking.

Ingredients:
- ¾ cup sliced almonds (blanched or unbalanced)
- ¼ cup all-purpose flour
- 10 tablespoons granulated sugar
- 3 tablespoons orange juice (freshly squeezed)
- 3 tablespoons butter (salted or unsalted)
- 2 tablespoons white sesame seeds
- 1 tablespoon toasted sesame oil
- 1½ teaspoons black sesame seeds
- Zest of 1 orange

Method:
1. Warm the sesame oil, butter, sugar, orange juice and orange zest in a small saucepan over a low heat until all the ingredients have melted and are smooth.
2. Remove from the heat and stir in the almonds, sesame seeds and flour.
3. Let this rest for 1 hour at room temperature.
4. Preheat your oven to 375F and line two baking sheets with parchment paper.
5. Drop a tablespoon (level) of batter, evenly spaced, on each baking sheet with four per sheet. Dampen your fingers and flatten the batter a little.
6. Bake in the oven, one sheet at a time is best, for 8 to 9 minutes until the cookies are evenly browned. Rotate the baking sheet halfway through baking.
7. Remove from oven, leave to cool for 1 minute.
8. Using a spatula (metal is best) lift each cookie off of the baking sheet and drape it over a rolling pin so it forms a curve. If the cookies are too hard to shape then put them in the oven for half a minute or so to soften them.

9. Once they have cooled on the rolling pin, remove the tuiles and place on a wire rack.
10. Repeat with the rest of the batter.

Red Grape Cake

This is an Italian style cake that is juicy and tasty with the roasted grapes in it. The cake can be wrapped in plastic wrap and stored at room temperature for no more than 3 days if you cannot manage all of the cake in one sitting. The cake goes very well with a sweet Italian wine or with small glasses of grappa. This recipe will make a cake large enough for 8 to 10 servings.

Note that if you add all the grapes at once you can find that they all sink to the bottom. If you reserve half the grapes and then bake the cake for 10 minutes before adding the rest of the grapes they will be in the top half of the cake.

Ingredients:
- 2 eggs
- 10oz red seedless grapes (washed and dried)
- 1 cup all-purpose flour (unbleached)
- 2/3 cup granulated sugar
- ½ cup yellow cornmeal
- ½ cup extra-virgin olive oil
- 1/3 cup milk
- 1½ teaspoon baking powder
- 1 teaspoon lemon zest (grated)
- 1 teaspoon pure vanilla extract
- ¼ teaspoon salt
- Confectioners' sugar (for dusting the cake before serving)

Method:
1. Preheat your oven to 350F and grease a 9" round spring form pan.
2. In a medium bowl whisk together the salt, baking powder, flour and cornmeal.
3. In a large mixing bowl, combine the sugar and eggs and beat for about 5 minutes with an electric beater until it increases in volume and is lighter in color.
4. Turn the mixer to a low setting and slowly but steadily add the oil.
5. Turn the mixer up to medium and beat for a further minute.
6. Mix in the lemon zest, vanilla and milk, beating on a low speed.
7. With the mixer on a low speed add the flour mixture ½ a cup at a time until just mixed.
8. Stir in half the grapes and then scrape the batter into the prepared pan and bake in the oven for 10 minutes.
9. Scatter the rest of the grapes on top of the cake and bake for about 40 minutes more until the cake is golden and a toothpick inserted in to the middle of the cake comes out clean.
10. Transfer the pan to a wire rack and cool for 5 minutes before releasing the sides from the pan and leaving to cool.
11. Dust with confectioners' sugar and cut in to wedges to serve.

Orange And Hazelnut Cookies

These cookies are very similar to biscotti and are not too sweet. They are ideal for dipping in coffee after a meal or as a snack by themselves. You can make the dough in advance and freeze it for up to a month. This recipe will make 72 cookies!

Ingredients:
- 10oz all-purpose flour (unbleached)
- 2 eggs
- 2 cups hazelnuts (toasted and skinned)
- ¾ cup plus 2 tablespoons granulated sugar
- ½ cup extra-virgin olive oil
- 1 teaspoon pure vanilla extract
- 1 teaspoon baking powder
- ¼ teaspoon table salt
- Zest of 2 medium sized oranges

Method:
1. Finely grind the hazelnuts in your food processor.
2. In a medium bowl mix together the salt, baking powder, hazelnuts and flour.
3. In a separate bowl, using a hand mixer (or stand mixer with paddle attachment) beat the eggs, zest, vanilla, oil and sugar on a low speed for about 15 seconds until the sugar is damp.
4. Then, on a high speed, mix for a further 15 seconds until well combined.
5. Add the dry ingredients and mix, on a low speed, for between 30 and 60 seconds until the dough has pulled together.
6. Divide the dough in two and put one half on to a piece of parchment paper. Shape the dough into an 11" long, 2" wide log. Wrap the parchment around the log and twist the ends to secure.
7. Repeat the previous step with the other piece of dough then chill both pieces in your freezer for an hour or until firm.
8. Preheat your oven to 350F and place two racks in the oven; one in the top third and one in the bottom half. Line four cookie sheets with parchment paper.
9. Take one dough log at a time and cut it into ¼" slices and place them 1" apart on the prepared sheets.
10. Bake 2 sheets at a time until golden on the bottom and edges. This will take about 10 minutes. Rotate and swap the sheets halfway through the cooking.
11. Allow to cool on racks and store in an airtight container, where they will keep for up to a week at room temperature.

Nutty Baklava

This is an interesting variation on baklava, a classic Greek dessert. It has a delicious tart citrus taste that goes well with the sweet and flaky layers. This dish is at its best 24 hours after you have added the syrup and it will keep for up to 5 days at room temperature, though it will become more crystalized and solid as more time passes. This recipe will make 30 pieces of baklava.

Ingredients:
- 2 x 8oz packs of phyllo dough (around twenty 9x14" sheets)
- 12oz dried apricots
- 12oz raw pistachios (unsalted and shelled)
- 10oz unsalted butter
- ½ cup granulated sugar
- 1½ cups granulated sugar
- 2/3 cup orange juice (freshly squeezed is best)
- 1½ teaspoons ground cardamom

Method:
1. Thaw the pastry overnight in your refrigerator and then leave at room temperature for about 2 hours before use.
2. Blend the pistachios, ½ cup of sugar and apricots in your food processor (in batches if necessary) for around 45 seconds until the nuts are finely chopped – about the size of dried lentils is best and then put to one side.
3. Unfold one of the pastry packs and stack them on top of each other so they lie flat on your counter top. Cover them loosely with plastic wrap, letting it fall down the four sides. Dampen some kitchen towel and wring it out so it is not sodden and drape it over the plastic wrap to prevent the pastry from drying out.
4. Melt the butter in a small saucepan and use some of it to brush the bottom of a 9x13" metal pan (straight sides are best).
5. Remove one sheet of pastry from the stack (re-cover the stack afterwards) and place it in the bottom of the pan.
6. Brush the sheet with melted butter, but do not soak it.
7. Repeat this until you have used half the first pack (about 10 sheets).
8. Sprinkle a third of the filling over the pastry making sure it is evenly spread.
9. Repeat the layering and buttering process for the rest of the pastry sheets in the first pack and then cover with another third of the filling.
10. Repeat the process again with the second pack of pastry, ending up with a final layer of pastry.
11. Cover loosely and leave it in the freezer for half an hour.
12. Preheat your oven to 350F and place an oven rack in the middle of your oven.
13. Before the baklava goes in to the oven, cut it diagonally with a sharp, serrated knife using a sawing motion at 1½ to 2 inch intervals. This allows the syrup to spread throughout the baklava and determines portion size. Avoid pressing down on the pastry and compressing it.
14. Bake in the oven for 45 minutes or until golden and then transfer to a cooling rack to cool.
15. Run a knife again along the cuts to help the syrup absorb more evenly.
16. In a small saucepan, bring the orange juice and sugar to a simmer, stirring occasionally until the liquid is clear and the sugar dissolved (around 5 minutes).
17. Remove from the heat and stir in the cardamom.
18. Pour this syrup evenly over the baklava so it runs down the cut marks and along the sides of the pan.
19. Leave to cool to room temperature before serving.

There are numerous variations on the baklava recipe, all of which follow the same process with just a few minor changes in ingredients.

Classic Baklava

Makes around 30 pieces.

Filling Ingredients:
- 1lb raw pistachios or almonds (shelled and unsalted)
- 10oz unsalted butter
- ½ cup granulated sugar
- 1 teaspoon ground cardamom
- 1 teaspoon ground cinnamon

Syrup Ingredients:
- 1½ cups granulated sugar
- 1½ teaspoons orange flower water

Pastry:
- 2 x 8oz packs of phyllo dough

The method is exactly the same as the previous recipe.

As some variations you can blend the nuts with dried fruit, chocolate liqueur and espresso which make for some interesting and tasty variations.

Hazelnut And Chocolate Baklava

This recipe follows the same method as the previous baklava recipes and will make around 30 pieces.

Filling Ingredients:
- 1lb raw hazelnuts (shelled)
- 10oz unsalted butter
- 6 oz bittersweet or semisweet chocolate (coarsely chopped)
- ¼ cup granulated sugar
- 2 teaspoons ground cardamom

Syrup Ingredients:
- 1½ cups granulated sugar
- 2 tablespoons Frangelico
- 2 teaspoons instant espresso powder

Pastry:
- 2 x 8oz packs of phyllo dough

Rosemary Cornmeal Cake

This is an interesting cake that goes down well at dinner parties. You can bake this cake the day before, brush it with syrup and then let it cool before wrapping it in plastic wrap and storing overnight. Then the next afternoon you can glaze the cake ready for serving. This recipe will make a cake that will produce 8 to 10 servings.

Cake Ingredients:
- 10oz granulated sugar
- 5oz mascarpone (at room temperature)
- 4 eggs
- 1½ cups all-purpose flour
- ¾ cup yellow cornmeal (finely ground)
- ½ cup unsalted butter (melted)
- 1/3 cup toasted pine nuts (coarsely chopped)
- 1 tablespoon orange zest (finely grated)
- 1 tablespoon fresh rosemary (finely chopped)
- 1 teaspoon baking powder
- ¼ teaspoon salt

Orange Syrup Ingredients:
- ½ cup fresh orange juice
- 3 tablespoons granulated sugar

Orange Glaze Ingredients:
- 5oz confectioners' sugar (sifted)
- 5 tablespoons heavy cream
- 2 tablespoons fresh orange juice
- 1 tablespoon fresh rosemary leaves (whole and stripped from the stem)
- 1 teaspoon grated orange zest

Cake Method:
1. Preheat your oven to 350F and place a rack in the middle of the oven.
2. Butter a 9x20" round cake pan and line the bottom with a circle of parchment paper. Use some softened butter to grease this.
3. In a medium bowl mix together the cornmeal, flour, rosemary, pine nuts, orange zest, salt and baking powder, ensuring it is well mixed.
4. Put the mascarpone in a large bowl and give it a quick whisk to loosen it up.
5. Add the eggs, one at a time, whisking after each one to combine.
6. Add the sugar and whisk until the mixture becomes smooth.
7. Using a rubber spatula, fold the dry ingredients in to the wet ingredients in two batches and mix until smooth.
8. Stir in the melted butter and mix until blended.
9. Pour the batter in to the prepared pan and spread evenly.
10. Bake for between 40 and 45 minutes until the top is a golden brown color and springs back when pressed. A toothpick pushed into the middle of the cake should come out looking a little bit moist.

Orange Syrup Method:
1. Heat the sugar and orange juice in a small saucepan, stirring occasionally, over a medium heat for 4 or 5 minutes until the sugar has dissolved.
2. Allow the cake to cool for 5 minutes in the pan and then run a small knife around the outside of the cake (between the cake and the pan wall). Place a plate upside down over the cake pan and turn the whole thing upside down (careful as the pan is going to be hot so protect your hands). The cake will slide out on to the plate.
3. Remove the parchment paper and place another inverted plate over the cake and turn the whole thing upside down so the cake is the right way round. Remove the top plate.
4. Use a skewer or toothpick and poke several dozen holes in the top of the cake.
5. Whilst the cake is warm, brush it with the syrup and keep brushing it for a few minutes to allow the syrup to sink in to the cake. Keep going until all the syrup is used up and then let the cake cool fully.

Orange Glaze Method:
1. Boil a small saucepan of water and prepare a bowl of ice water.
2. Put the rosemary leaves in a sieve and then dip it into the boiling water for 1 minute to blanch them. Remove them from the water, shake to get off excess water and place immediately in the bowl of ice water (still in the sieve). Drain the leaves and then spread on to a paper towel and allow to dry.
3. Whisk together in a bowl the cream, confectioners' sugar and orange juice until smooth.
4. Mix in the rosemary and zest and ensure well combined.
5. Once the cake is cool, place a baking sheet below the wire rack and transfer your cake on to a cardboard round.
6. Pour the glaze over the top of the cake, allowing it to drip over the sides.
7. Before the glaze dries, transfer the cake to a cake plate.
8. Leave to sit for an hour before cutting and serving.

Honey Spiced Walnut Tart

Another interesting dessert that will definitely impress! This can be made earlier in the day and then heated in a hot oven for a few minutes before serving. The recipe will make a tart large enough to serve 8 to 10 people.

Ingredients:
- 1 sheet (9oz) frozen puff pastry (thawed)
- 1 egg
- 1 cup walnuts (roughly chopped)
- 1/3 cup honey
- 4 tablespoons unsalted butter (slightly softened)
- 2 tablespoons granulated sugar
- 1½ teaspoons ground cinnamon
- 1 teaspoon ground ginger
- Pinch of salt

Method:
1. Preheat your oven to 400F.
2. Blend together the salt, ginger, sugar, honey, cinnamon and butter either in a food processor or using a bowl and spoon.
3. Add the egg and beat until blended.
4. Add the nuts and blend thoroughly. Be careful in a food processor that the nuts are not blended smooth as you want a crunch from them.
5. Cut the pastry sheet in half and roll one strip to be 15"x6" in size.
6. Prick the whole surface with a fork and then slide the sheet on to a baking sheet lined with parchment paper.
7. Spread the nut mixture on the pastry to within ½" of the long edges and all the way to the short edges.
8. Fold the ½" bare pastry over the nut mixture and press firmly to stick. Crimp the edges of the pastry.
9. Repeat this with the second pastry strip and the remaining nut mixture on a second baking tray.
10. Bake for around 20 minutes until the filling starts to look a little dry on top and the pastry has turned a deep golden brown color.
11. Cool slightly before serving and cut each tart in to 4 or 5 strips.

MEDITERRANEAN SNACK RECIPES

Snacks are probably the hardest part of any healthy eating program. When you need to snack the temptation is to grab a chocolate bar or other unhealthy snack because they are convenient and provide a quick sugar boost. The key is to have alternatives to hand that are healthy and that you can quickly grab without having to take a lot of time to prepare it.

This section will detail some very healthy snack recipes that are pretty easy to make. Many of these can be made in advance and stored for use when you need them. The dips and hummus are great with some sliced vegetables such as bell peppers, cucumber, carrot and celery or even with the baked sweet potato fries detailed below.

I would recommend making several of these dishes and then storing them for use during the following few days. It means that when you want a healthy snack there is one there ready and waiting for you and the temptation to eat junk food will be so much lower.

There are plenty of snacks that you can have that do not require any preparation at all. These are great for when you are on the go as you can often find these in the stores, meaning you can get a diet friendly snack whilst out and about.

Kumquats are a very tart citrusy fruit, like a small orange though you eat the rind and seeds. About 7 kumquats will give you your entire recommended daily allowance of Vitamin C, a good amount of vitamin A plus iron and calcium! They are not messy to eat, making them an ideal snack for on the go and can be eaten alone or added to a salad with goat cheese, dried cranberries, nuts and chopped apples!

Plain Greek yogurt is another healthy snack with a rich and tangy taste. It can be eaten as is or through in some fresh or dried fruit for a more interested snack. Greek yogurt is high in protein with a 6oz serving having as much as 18g of protein, which is equivalent to eating 3 eggs, but without the unhealthy fats.

Another good snack is dried apples, either store bought (always choose the unsweetened variety) or home-made. These will help to reduce your bad cholesterol levels and give you some good fiber. The also contain polyphenols which are a group of chemicals which not only affect how your body produces cholesterol but also affects the fat around your middle. You can make your own by thinly slicing some apples, arranging them on a cookie sheet (sprinkle with cinnamon for a special treat) and bake for around 2 hours at 200F. Keep a close eye on them as they can burn.

Pistachio nuts are a great snack, having the lowest calorie count of all the nuts. A 1oz serving, which is around 50 nuts, contains only 160 calories! It is also packed with the healthy antioxidants found in almonds and walnuts. Because you typically buy pistachios in their shell, they take a while to eat, which makes you feel fuller and discourages over eating.

Medjool dates are a seriously sweet treat that will give you your sugar fix! They are sticky, tender and absolutely delicious though a couple of dates will give you around 140 calories! Whilst they are high in sugar they are also high in antioxidants and do not appear to have any negative affect on your blood sugar levels according to scientific studies.

Another great and handy snack is pumpkin seeds which contain tryptophan, an amino acid used by the body to create serotonin. You can roast your own or buy them already roasted. Simple spread them on a baking sheet, drizzle with olive oil, season with salt and pepper and roast for 15 minutes at 350F, stirring occasionally. These can also be used in salads or in yogurt as well as being eaten as is.

Roasted Chickpeas

This is a great snack that is high in healthy mono-unsaturated fats and delicious. They can be eaten warm or stored and eaten over the next few days. They dip well in to hummus or other dips and are surprisingly tasty.

Ingredients:
- 2 cans of chickpeas (rinsed, drained and patted dry)
- 2 tablespoons olive oil
- Paprika – to taste
- Salt – to taste

Method:
1. Place the chickpeas on a rimmed baking tray and drizzle the olive oil over them. Toss them well to ensure the oil coats them all.
2. Bake in a hot oven for between 30 to 40 minutes until dark and crunchy.
3. Remove from the oven, sprinkle the salt and paprika over them and stir well.
4. Cook for another 4 to 5 minutes and then remove from the oven and cool.

Baked Sweet Potato Fries

Another heart healthy snack using one of the healthiest and most beneficial vegetables there are! Sweet potatoes are absolutely loaded with the antioxidant carotenoid which will help lower you risk of a wide variety of diseases. They are also full of fiber, meaning they have a low glycemic index, and are extremely tasty! These can be dipped in hummus or one of the other dips in this section or served as they are. Store in an air tight container and eat within 2 or 3 days.

Ingredients:
- 2 tablespoons olive oil
- 3 or 4 sweet potatoes
- Salt and pepper to taste
- Optional – basil, paprika or cayenne pepper

Method:
1. Preheat your oven to 425F.
2. Slice the potatoes lengthwise into ½" fries and then toss in a bowl with the olive oil
3. Season to taste and add any other spices you like and then toss again.
4. Lay out in a single layer on a rimmed baking tray.
5. Bake for 30 minutes, turning them every 10 minutes.

Banana Gelato

This is a great snack for when you need something sweet! It is easy to make and can be eaten as is or spread on graham crackers.

Ingredients:
- 2 bananas

Method:
1. Peel the bananas and slice them.
2. Place them on a cookie sheet in a single layer and freeze for 2 hours.
3. Blend in your food processor until it has a smooth consistency and serve immediately.

Make this more interesting by adding peanut or hazelnut butter or fresh berries for some extra taste!

Hummus

This recipe will make around 5 cups of hummus and is the type traditionally found in the West. It is easy to make and will keep for a few days in your refrigerator. It makes for a great snack when served with pitta bread or sliced fresh vegetables.

Ingredients:
- 2 x 15oz cans garbanzo beans (drained)
- 6 garlic cloves (peeled and crushed)
- 4 tablespoons lemon juice
- 3 tablespoons tahini
- ¼ teaspoon crushed red pepper flakes

Method:
1. Blend the beans in your food processor until they become a spreadable paste.
2. Add the rest of the ingredients and blend until smooth, adding more lemon juice if you feel the consistency is too thick.

Traditional Hummus

This is a more traditional hummus recipe and is slightly different from the above. It will make about 2½ cups of hummus.

Ingredients:
- 19oz can garbanzo beans (reserve half the liquid, discard the rest)
- 1 garlic clove (chopped)
- 4 tablespoons lemon juice
- 2 tablespoons olive oil
- 2 tablespoons tahini
- 1 teaspoon salt
- Black pepper to taste

Method:
1. Add the beans and reserved juice to the blender, keeping a tablespoon of the whole beans to one side.
2. Add the salt, garlic, tahini and lemon juice and blend until creamy and thoroughly mixed.
3. Transfer the hummus to a serving bowl and sprinkle with pepper.
4. Pour the olive oil over the top and garnish with the reserved beans.

Black Bean Hummus

This is a good variation of the hummus recipe which will make around 8 servings. It uses black beans and olives to give the hummus a bit of extra taste.

Ingredients:
- 15oz can black beans (drain but reserve the liquid)
- 1 garlic clove (minced)
- 10 Greek olives
- 2 tablespoons lemon juice
- 1½ tablespoons tahini
- ¾ teaspoon ground cumin
- ½ teaspoon salt
- ¼ teaspoon paprika
- Pinch of cayenne pepper

Method:
1. Put the black beans, 2 tablespoons of their liquid, lemon juice, cumin, salt, cayenne pepper and tahini in to your food process and blend until smooth (scrape down the sides of the blender as needed).
2. Add any additional seasoning or liquid to get the right consistency and taste for you.
3. Turn out in to a bowl and garnish with Greek olives and paprika.

Roasted Red Pepper Hummus

This has to be my favorite hummus and you can make your own roasted red peppers rather than buying them if you prefer (drizzle them with olive oil and cook in your oven until they start to char). This is a really tasty hummus that goes very well with sliced fresh vegetables. This recipe will make enough for around 8 servings.

Ingredients:
- 15oz can garbanzo beans (drained)
- 4oz jar roasted red peppers
- 1 garlic clove (minced)
- 3 tablespoons lemon juice
- 1½ tablespoons tahini
- 1 tablespoon fresh parsley (chopped)
- ½ teaspoon cayenne pepper
- ½ teaspoon ground cumin
- ¼ teaspoon salt

Method:
1. Add all the ingredients, except the parsley, to your food process and blend, using pulses, until the mixture is smooth and slightly fluffy (scrape the mixture off the sides as required).
2. Transfer the hummus to a bowl and refrigerate for an hour before serving garnished with the parsley.

Grape Leaf Aleppo

This is a great snack for the day and can be stored in your refrigerator for up to 3 days. They can also be served as a starter for a meal or as a side. This recipe makes 32 servings.

Ingredients:
- 2 x 16oz jars grape leaves (drained and rinsed)
- 2lbs ground lamb
- 6 garlic cloves (sliced)
- 2 Kalamata olives
- 1 cup lemon juice
- 1 cup white rice (uncooked)
- 1 tablespoon ground allspice
- 1 teaspoon ground black pepper
- 1 teaspoon salt

Method:
1. Soak the rice in cold water and then drain.
2. Mix in a large bowl the rice, lamb, salt, pepper and allspice until well mixed.
3. Place a tablespoon of this mixture in to the middle of each grape leaf.
4. Fold the leaf over once, turn in the edges on each side and roll the leaf closed.
5. Stack the rolls in a large pot with each layer covered in slices of garlic. Do not stack higher than 3 or 4 rolls as they can cook unevenly. Use a second saucepan if necessary or cook in two batches.
6. Add enough water to cover the leaf rolls and then add the lemon juice and olives (to give flavor).
7. Place a small plate on top of the rolls so they stay underwater and bring the pan to the boil.
8. Reduce the heat, cover the pan and simmer for 1¼ hours.
9. Taste the rice to ensure it is done and then remove, carefully from the water. These are best left to sit for several hours to get more flavor.

Tzatziki Sauce

This is a very traditional Greek sauce that is very delicious. It can be served on the side for all sorts of meals or eaten with fresh vegetables or pita bread as a dip. This recipe will make around 1½ cups of taztziki. This will store for a couple of days in your refrigerator.

Ingredients:
- 8oz plain yogurt
- 3 cloves garlic (pressed)
- 2 tablespoons olive oil
- 1 tablespoon fresh dill (chopped)
- 1 tablespoon lemon juice
- ½ teaspoon each of salt and pepper

Method:
1. Blend together all of the ingredients in your food processor until well combined and then serve.

Feta Garlic Dip

Another simple to make dip that will store for a couple of days in your refrigerator. This recipe will make 1 cup of dip and can be used with fresh vegetables or pita bread.

Ingredients:
- 2 garlic cloves (peeled)
- 1 cup feta cheese (crumbled)
- ½ cup plain yogurt
- ½ cup sour cream
- ¼ teaspoon each salt and pepper

Method:
1. Put all the ingredients (except the salt and pepper) into your food processor and blend until the garlic is well minced.
2. Pour into a serving bowl and season with the salt and pepper.

Avocado Tzatziki

A good variation of the traditional taztziki that includes the wonder health fruit, the avocado. It makes for a very interesting taste and can be served as a side or eaten with sliced fresh vegetables or pita bread. This recipe makes enough for 8 people.

Ingredients:
- 1 avocado (peeled and pitted)
- 2 garlic cloves (minced)
- Juice of 1 lemon
- ½ cup cucumber (chopped and deseeded)
- ¼ cup sour cream
- 1 tablespoon fresh cilantro (chopped)
- 1 tablespoon fresh mint (chopped)
- ½ teaspoon red pepper flakes

Method:
1. Mix together the garlic, avocado, sour cream, cucumber and lemon juice in a food processor and blend until smooth (if your avocado is ripe then you can mash this all together in a bowl).
2. Season with cilantro, mint, red pepper flakes and salt and pepper (to taste) and mix well.
3. Cover and refrigerate for an hour before serving.

Roasted Red Pepper Feta Dip

This is another great dip that can be used like the others for a snack. It is quick and easy to make and very tasty. You can roast the bell pepper at home yourself or buy a jar or roasted red peppers and use the equivalent. This recipe makes about 1¾ cups of dip.

Ingredients:
- 8oz feta cheese
- 1 red bell pepper (roasted – though you can use jarred peppers)
- 1 garlic clove (minced)
- ¼ cup plain yogurt
- Pinch of cayenne pepper

Method:
1. Add all the ingredients to your food processor and blend until smooth.

Halloumi Cheese Fingers

These make a great snack but can be served with a Greek salad and some warm crusty bread for a great lunch. This recipe makes enough for 2 servings.

Ingredients:
- 6oz halloumi cheese (cut into ½" sticks)
- ½ tablespoon extra-virgin olive oil
- 2 teaspoons fresh lemon juice
- ¼ teaspoon dried oregano

Method:
1. Heat the oil in a frying pan on a medium heat (alternatively you can grill the cheese if you prefer brushed in olive oil) for 1 or 2 minutes until the cheese turns a light golden brown color.
2. Sprinkle with lemon juice, oregano and season with pepper before serving.

Taramousalata

This is a dish that will definitely impress guests as it is also known as "Greek caviar". Any leftovers will freeze and can be thawed and used when required. It is served chilled with either pita or crusty bread. The recipe will make around 3½ cups.

Ingredients:
- 8 slices white sandwich bread
- 1 potato
- 1 small onion (chopped)
- 2 Greek olives
- 2 cups milk
- ½ cup extra-virgin olive oil
- ½ cup carp roe
- ¼ cup fresh lemon juice

Method:
1. Preheat your oven to 450F.
2. Wash the potato and prick it several times with a fork. Place on a baking sheet and cook for around an hour until a knife easily goes through it.
3. Cool then peel and chop.
4. Place the bread in to a shallow dish and cover with the milk. Leave to soak for 5 minutes then squeeze the milk out of the bread. Keep the bread and discard the milk.
5. Add all the ingredients except the olives) to your food processor and blend for around 60 seconds until fluffy. Add more olive oil if necessary to get the right consistency.
6. Turn out in to a bowl, chill and garnish with the Greek olives before serving.

MEDITERRANEAN BREAD RECIPES

Breads are a big part of the Mediterranean diet and many meals are served with a good sized chunk of bread. The difference is that the Mediterranean breads are home-made, healthy and full of goodness for you, not having the processed flour and chemicals in that many of our Western breads contain.

With the majority of these recipes you can use a bread maker on a dough cycle for kneading and rising the dough. If so then follow the manufacturer's instructions and adjust the recipe as appropriate.

These breads make an ideal accompaniment to many of the other recipes detailed in this book or can be used as a snack with one of the many dips you can make.

Black Olive Bread

This is a really delicious bread and you can use any type of olive you like with it from the traditional black olives to Kalamata or even green. Some people like to add some sun-dried tomatoes to the recipe to give it some extra taste.

Ingredients:
- 3 cups bread flour
- 1¼ cups warm water (110F)
- ½ cup black olives (chopped)
- 3 tablespoons olive oil
- 2 tablespoons white sugar
- 1 tablespoon cornmeal
- 2 teaspoons active dry yeast
- 1 teaspoons salt

Method:
1. In a large bowl mix together the flour, yeast, salt, olives, sugar, water and olive oil.
2. Turn this dough out on to a floured surface and knead for 5 to 10 minutes until smooth and elastic.
3. Leave for 45 minutes in a warm place to rise until it has doubled in size.
4. Punch down and knead for a further 5 to 10 minutes.
5. Leave again in a warm place for a further 30 minutes until doubled in size.
6. Round the dough on a floured surface and then place upside down in an oiled glass bowl. Leave in a warm place until it has doubled in size.
7. Put a pan of water in the bottom of your oven and preheat to 500F.
8. Careful turn the loaf out on to a lightly oiled sheet pan (dust the pan with the cornmeal).
9. Bake for 15 minutes at 500F and then reduce the heat to 375F and cook for a further 30 minutes.

Mozzarella Bruschetta

This is a great snack, starter or side where the bruschetta is topped with a delicious pepper mix. The topping can be adjusted as you wish with a wide variety of options available to you.

Ingredients:
- 3½oz Mozzarella cheese (thinly sliced)
- 8 sliced ciabatta bread
- 16 black olives
- 1 red bell pepper (deseeded and cut into thin strips)
- 2oz butter
- 1 tablespoon lemon juice
- 1 tablespoon fresh parsley or rosemary
- Pinch of sugar

Method:
1. Heat the butter in a frying pan and sauté the peppers, herbs and sugar. Cover and cook on a medium heat for 20 minutes, stirring occasionally. The peppers should be soft but not brown.
2. Stir in the lemon juice.
3. Grill the bread slices until both sides are golden brown but the bread is still chewy.
4. Place some pepper mixture on to the toast, top with 2 olives and some cheese.
5. Grill for a minute or two until the cheese has melted and then serve immediately.

Sun Dried Tomato Scones

This recipe will make 12 delicious savory scones which are a great compliment to soups or can even be spread with one of the many dips detailed earlier.

Ingredients:
- 6oz self raising flour
- 3oz feta cheese (cut into small cubes)
- 2oz feta cheese (crumbled)
- 2oz whole wheat flour
- 2oz sun dried tomatoes (chopped and drained but reserve 1 tablespoon of oil)
- 10 black olives (roughly chopped)
- 1 large egg
- 2 tablespoons extra-virgin olive oil
- 2 tablespoons milk
- 1½ teaspoons fresh thyme (chopped)
- ¼ teaspoon baking powder
- ¼ teaspoon mustard powder
- ¼ teaspoon cayenne pepper
- Milk for brushing

Method:
1. Sift the baking powder and flour in to a large bowl, tipping anything left in the sieve in to the bowl.
2. Add the mustard powder and cayenne pepper.
3. Use a knife and work in 2 tablespoons of olive oil plus the reserved tablespoon of oil from the sun-dried tomatoes.
4. Once the mixture is looking like lumpy breadcrumbs then you can stir in the cubed feta, sun dried tomatoes, chopped thyme and olives.
5. In a separate bowl beat the egg together with 2 tablespoons of milk.
6. Add half of this to the other mixture and use your hands to bring the mixture together to form a dough, adding more of the egg and milk mixture as required. You are aiming for a soft dough that is not sticky.
7. Roll the dough out on a floured surface so it is 1" thick.
8. Using a 2" cutter, cut out the scones which are then put on a baking tray. Re-roll any remaining pastry and cut out more scones. Brush each scone with milk.
9. Top each scone with some crumbled feta cheese.
10. Put the tray on the highest shelf in your oven and cook until they turn a golden color, around 12 to 15 minutes.
11. Remove from the heat, cool on a wire rack and serve.

Focaccia Bread

This is a traditional Italian bread that goes well with many of the meals detailed previously in this book. Instead of using plain olive oil in this recipe try olive oil infused with basil or even chilli to give the bread an extra special taste.

Ingredients:
- 5 cups all-purpose flour (plus extra for kneading)
- 1¾ cups warm water
- 1 cup extra-virgin olive oil (divided)
- 1 tablespoon sugar
- 1 tablespoon salt
- 1 package active dry yeast
- Coarse sea salt (for sprinkling)

Method:
1. In a small bowl mix together the yeast, sugar and warm water. Put the bowl in a warm place for at least 15 minutes until the yeast is fragrant and bubbling.
2. Put the dough hook on your mixer and mix the flour, ½ cup of olive oil, yeast mixture and salt on a low speed. Knead for another 5 minutes on a medium speed when the dough has come together until it becomes smooth and soft. If it becomes too sticky, sprinkle some more flour on it.
3. Knead the dough on a floured surface a few times, sprinkling with more flour if it is too sticky.
4. Coat the inside of a glass bowl with olive oil, put the dough in the bowl, cover with plastic wrap and leave for an hour in a warm place until doubled in size.
5. Coat a jelly roll pan with ½ cup of olive oil – remember focaccia is an oily bread which gives it its taste.
6. Turn the dough out in to the jelly roll pan and press it down so it fits in the pan properly, turning the dough over so it is thoroughly coated in olive oil.
7. Continue stretching the dough out to fill the pan and make finger holes down into the dough which will give it the crusty, craggy look that makes focaccia so distinctive.
8. Place the dough in a warm place for an hour until it has doubled in size.
9. Preheat your oven to 425F.
10. Sprinkle the top of the bread with coarse sea salt and drizzle some olive oil over it. Note that you can also sprinkle rosemary, parsley, basil, chopped olives or other herbs on top if you would like. You can also place some chopped tomatoes on the top of the bread 5 minutes before it is cooked to give it a sun blushed look.
11. Bake the bread for 25-30 minutes until the top is golden brown then remove from the oven and allow to cool before serving.

Whole Wheat Pita Bread

This is a simple recipe for making your own pita bread which can be used for many of the dishes you have learned to cook, including being cut in to strips and served with one of the many tasty dips as a treat. This recipe will make 8 pita breads.

Ingredients:
- 10oz bread flour
- 4¾oz whole wheat flour
- 1 cup warm water (about 100F)
- 2 tablespoons light sour cream
- 1 tablespoon extra-virgin olive oil
- 1 tablespoon sugar
- 2¼ teaspoons instant yeast
- ¾ teaspoon salt
- Cornmeal

Method:
1. Mix the sugar, yeast and ½ a cup of water in the bowl of a stand mixer.
2. In a medium bowl whisk together the flours and add ½ cup of this mixture to the yeast. Whisk until smooth.
3. Cover the mixer bowl with plastic wrap and leave somewhere warm for around 45 minutes until bubbly and doubled in size.
4. Add the rest of the water and flour as well as the oil, salt and sour cream.
5. Using the dough hook on your mixer, mix on a low speed until the dough starts to come together (you may need to scrape down the sides).
6. Knead the dough for 5 minutes on a low speed until it is elastic and smooth.
7. Turn the dough out on to a floured work surface and shape it in a ball.
8. Oil a large bowl, put the dough in the bowl and cover with plastic wrap. Leave for an hour to rise, or until it has doubled in size.
9. Sprinkle two baking sheets with cornmeal and preheat your oven to 500F.
10. Turn the dough out on to a floured surface and cut into eight pieces of the same size.
11. Working on piece at a time, shape the piece of dough in to a ball then flatten to a disk.
12. Roll the dough into a 6" circle and transfer to the prepared baking sheets.
13. Repeat this with the rest of the dough pieces – note that you can find the dough springs back, in which case let it rest for a couple of minutes and roll it again.
14. Loosely cover the baking sheets with kitchen towel and leave to one side for 20 minutes until the dough becomes a little bit puffy.
15. Transfer a few pita breads at a time to your oven rack (in the middle of the oven) and bake for 2 minutes on each side, or until puffed up and golden in color.
16. Transfer the cooked pitas to a wire rack to cool and continue to all the pitas have been cooked.

Cheesy Sun-Dried Tomato Bread

This is a delicious bread that is full of flavor. You can add even more to it by adding some sliced olives, though that is optional.

Ingredients:

- 3 cups bread flour
- 1 cup water
- ¼ cup Parmesan cheese (grated)
- ¼ cup plain yogurt (fat free is best)
- 8 halves of sun-dried tomatoes
- 2 tablespoons sugar
- 1 tablespoon chopped fresh herbs (thyme, sage, oregano and rosemary all work well in this dish)
- 1½ teaspoons salt
- 1 package active dry yeast

Method:

1. Soak the sun-dried tomatoes in water for about 2 hours then drain well and pat dry with paper towels.
2. Heat the yogurt and water in a small saucepan until steaming, stirring to ensure it is well combined.
3. Remove from heat and leave to stand for around 5 minutes until it reaches between 120F and 130F.
4. Fit the dough hook to your stand mixer and add to the bowl half the flour, yeast, cheese, herbs, sugar and salt. Mix it well.
5. Add the yogurt mixture and ensure it is well combined.
6. Add the tomatoes and mix again.
7. Add the rest of the flour, a quarter of a cup at a time, mixing on a low speed until the dough is tacky when touched and clears the bowl. Note that you may not need all of the flour and you can save or discard whatever is left.
8. Knead on a medium speed for 6 or 7 minutes until it is elastic and smooth.
9. Grease a bowl, put the dough in and cover with a plastic wrap. Leave in a warm place for around an hour until doubled in size.
10. Punch down the dough and knead it a few times.
11. Roll the dough gently in to a 7x14" rectangle (roughly).
12. Starting on the short side, tightly roll the dough up. Pinch the ends together to seal the roll and then tuck the ends underneath.
13. Place in a greased 9x5" loaf pan and cover with plastic wrap. Let it rise until when you press it with your finger it leaves an indentation.
14. Preheat your oven to 350F.
15. Bake for around 30 minutes until golden brown then remove from oven and leave to cool for 10 minutes in the pan before turning it out on to a wire rack to cool.

Ciabatta Bread

This is a very traditional Italian bread made with olive oil which is great to make. It is a simple bread to make and this recipe will make 2 loaves.

Ingredients:
- 3¼ cups bread flour
- 1½ cups water
- 1 tablespoon olive oil
- 1½ teaspoons salt
- 1½ teaspoons bread machine yeast
- 1 teaspoon white sugar

Method:
1. Put the ingredients in to the pan of your bread machine according to the manufacturer's instructions and select the dough cycle.
2. If you are using a stand mixer, add everything except the olive oil and mix on a low speed using a dough hook for 10 minutes before adding the olive oil and mixing for another 5 minutes.
3. The dough is going to be very sticky but do not add any more flour.
4. Place the dough on a well floured surface and cover with greased plastic wrap, allowing it to rest for 15 minutes.
5. Line two baking sheets with parchment paper or lightly flour them.
6. Using a serrated knife, cut the dough in to two pieces and shape in to a 3x14" oval.
7. Place the loaves in the prepared sheets and dust with flour.
8. Cover and leave in a warm place to rise for 45 minutes.
9. Preheat your oven to 425F.
10. Sprinkle some water over the loaves and place on the middle rack of your oven.
11. Bake for 25 to 30 minutes until golden brown.

Turkish Flat Bread

Known as bazlama locally, this is a delicious bread normally cooked in an outdoor oven, though can easily be cooked indoors on a conventional oven. This recipe will make 4 flatbreads which are best served warm. Any bread not eaten can be stored for up to 3 days in an airtight container. This can be used in similar ways to pita bread or eaten with soups or other meals.

Ingredients:
- 4 cups all-purpose flour
- 1½ cups warm water (110F/45C)
- ½ cup Greek yogurt
- 1 tablespoon salt
- 1 tablespoon white sugar
- ¼oz package active dry yeast

Method:
1. Dissolve the sugar, salt and yeast in the warm water.
2. Add the yogurt and water to the flour and mix thoroughly until it forms a soft dough that is not sticky.
3. Shape the dough into a ball on a lightly floured surface.
4. Cover the dough with a damp cloth and leave it for 3 hours at room temperature to rise.
5. Cut the dough into four and shape into rounds, flattening each one as if making pizza dough.
6. Cover with a damp cloth and let it rest for 15 minutes.
7. Heat a griddle or skillet over a medium to high heat and cook each dough round for about a minute on each side until the bottom starts to spot brown. Remove each piece of bread when done and keep warm in kitchen towel or in an oven, repeating until all dough rounds are cooked.
8. Serve warm or store in an airtight container.

Sun Dried Tomato Focaccia Bread

This is another delicious version of the popular focaccia bread which will go down well with anyone who loves the flavor of sun dried tomatoes. This recipe will make about six 5" focaccia breads using a bread machine.

Ingredients:
- 3 cups bread flour
- 1 cup Mozzarella cheese (shredded)
- 1 cup water
- ½ cup sun-dried tomatoes (chopped)
- 3½ tablespoons white sugar
- 3 tablespoons butter
- 2 tablespoons dry milk powder
- 2 tablespoons Parmesan Cheese
- 2 tablespoons extra-virgin olive oil
- 2 teaspoons active dry yeast
- 2 teaspoons dried rosemary (crushed)
- 1 teaspoon salt
- 1 teaspoon garlic salt
- Cornmeal (for dusting)

Method:
1. Put the flour, water, sugar, butter, salt, powdered milk and yeast in to your bread machine (follow the manufacturer's recommendations for the order) and start on a dough cycle. This should produce around ½lb of dough.
2. Knead the bread on a lightly floured surface for a minute and then place in an oiled bowl (turn to coat). Cover with a damp cloth and leave in a warm place for 15 minutes to rise.
3. Dust a 10x15" baking tray with cornmeal.
4. Roll the dough out so it fits in the pan then push your fingers in to the top of the dough to make small holes.

5. Brush the surface with oil, cover with a damp cloth and leave somewhere warm for 30 minutes to rise.
6. Sprinkle with the cheeses, rosemary and garlic salt.
7. Cook in an oven pre-heated to 400F for 15 minutes until it browns.
8. Allow it to cool a little before cutting in to squares and serving.

Parmesan Focaccia

This is a good variation on the focaccia bread that has a tasty cheesy tang to it. It is simple to make and uses a bread maker for the mixing and kneading, which you can do yourself if you prefer.

Ingredients:
- 4¼ cups bread flour
- 11 fluid ounces of water (warmed to 110F)
- 1/3 cup extra-virgin olive oil
- 1/3 cup Parmesan cheese (grated)
- 4 teaspoons extra-virgin olive oil
- 4 teaspoons dried oregano
- 3 teaspoons bread machine yeast
- 1 teaspoon lecithin
- 1 teaspoon salt
- 1 teaspoon white sugar

Method:
1. Put the ingredients (except the cheese and 4 teaspoons of olive oil) in to your bread machine in the order recommended by the manufacturer. Select the dough setting and start the machine.
2. Once the dough has risen, put it in an oiled 8" round baking tin.
3. Place somewhere warm and leave to rise until it has doubled in size.
4. Poke the surface with your finger to make holes all the way down to the bottom of the tin.
5. Leave to rest for 10 minutes.
6. Pour the olive oil over the top of the dough and sprinkle the cheese over the top.
7. Bake in an oven preheated to 400F for around 20 minutes until golden brown.

Lebanese Flatbread

This is a unique flatbread that has an interesting 'sultry' flavor that is great as an appetizer or can be served with a main course. The blend of spices is particularly interesting, though not overpowering. It can be served with hummus, olive oil or guacamole for dipping. Za'atar is a Lebanese spice which you may have to order online or obtain from a specialist shop, and it is worth spending the time to find it!

Ingredients:

- 2 cups all-purpose flour
- ¾ cup warm water (110F)
- ¼ cup extra-virgin olive oil
- ¼ cup extra-virgin olive oil (divided)
- ¼ cup Za'atar
- ¾ teaspoon salt
- ½ teaspoon salt
- ¼oz pack of active dry yeast

Method:

1. Mix the yeast and water in a large bowl and leave in a warm place for 10 minutes until a layer of foam appears.
2. Whisk in ¼ cup of olive oil before gradually stirring in the flour plus ½ teaspoon of salt.
3. On a lightly floured surface, knead the bread for around 10 minutes until it becomes smooth and slightly sticky.
4. Put the dough in an oiled bowl, turning to coat, and leave in your refrigerator overnight (it should double in size).
5. Coat a 9x13" baking sheet with 2 tablespoons of olive oil and put the dough in to the middle of the sheet, flattening it in to a thick disk.
6. Cover with plastic wrap and leave for about 90 minutes until doubled in size.
7. Press and stretch the dough out until it evenly fills the baking sheet.
8. Use your fingertips to make small indentations in the dough and brush with the remaining olive oil.
9. In a small bowl, stir in the ¾ teaspoon salt and Za'atar and sprinkle it over the dough.
10. Leave, uncovered, to rest for 30 minutes.
11. Bake in an over preheated to 375F for 15 to 20 minutes until golden brown in color.

THE MEDITERRANEAN DIET ON A BUDGET

You may be thinking that the Mediterranean Diet is going to cost you a lot of money and admittedly some of the components such as extra virgin olive oil are more expensive than sunflower or vegetable oil. However, the health benefits from these ingredients are significant and it is worth the money.

If you shop around some of the discount and bargain stores you can often find some of the key ingredients like olives, olive oil, pesto and whole wheat pasta at a much more attractive price.

The fresh produce can be found cheaply at farmer's markets or you can often find it on sale or reduced in the supermarkets. If you do find this produce cheap then you can prepare and freeze the excess, which is going to mean you have access to these vegetables when they are more expensive.

You can even prepare entire meals and then freeze them so they just need heating up when you need them. I tend to make a huge batch of pasta, soup or stew and then freeze most of it in portion sized containers (I have four freezers at home for this reason). Then I can heat it up when it is needed and I have a very healthy ready meal without the hassle of having to cook or prepare it.

Another good source of items for this diet is stores such as Costco or Makro. If you can join one of these then it will prove a huge money saver as you can get many of your cans and jars here at a good discount. You can also find a lot of fresh produce in bulk at good prices in these stores too. Many of the stores regularly run promotions on items which is a good time to stock up on them.

Couponing can be another great way to save money on your shopping. Look out for coupons for foods that are a part of your new eating program and collect them to get some great discounts. If you live in America then there are tons of coupons to collect and you can really stock your cupboards up for a fraction of the normal cost!

Shopping around, buying in bulk and even buying online will save you some money. You can even grow your own vegetables at home if you like, which can be a huge money saver. A packet of zucchini seeds will cost you a couple of bucks, if that, yet each plant will produce 20 to 30 delicious zucchini's! Growing your own vegetables is not too difficult and it is something you can do as a money saver if you are so inclined. If you are lacking in space then look at either vertical gardening, container gardening or square foot gardening, all of which are great ways for you to grow a lot of fresh produce in a relatively small area.

Buying direct from the source, i.e. from local farmers or growers is probably the cheapest way to get hold of fresh produce, though some ingredients like the extra-virgin olive oil are going to be more expensive. If you look around discount supermarkets you can usually find this oil at a much cheaper price than from a regular supermarket. Don't be tempted to buy virgin or just plain olive oil as this does not have the same benefits as extra-virgin olive oil, which is made from the first pressing of the olives.

There are a lot of options for you to save money on this diet and as you get used to the diet you will start shopping around. You will then work out which stores are the best for which items. I know my weekly shopping on this diet is done at six or seven different stores, including two market stalls (for fruit and vegetables) to ensure that I keep the costs right down and get good quality produce. If you are willing to spend that little bit of time shopping around you will be surprised how cheaply you can follow this diet.

The Mediterranean Diet can be a little bit more expensive than the normal junk food diet eaten by many people. However, you do have to think about what price to put on your health and wellbeing. From my own point of view I would rather go without my daily Starbuck's or newspaper and know that I am looking after myself so that I can live longer and see my children grow up.

WHAT TO EAT AND WHAT TO AVOID

For someone just starting out on this diet it can be very confusing as there are a lot of foods you can eat and lots that you need to avoid. Making the transition to the diet can be tricky but if you follow the advice in this book you are going to find it easy.

In this chapter we will discuss some of the foods you can buy and some of the ones you should avoid as they are harmful to you. Do not feel that you are overly limited on the Mediterranean Diet, it is one of the most varied and tasty diets out there and you will find that over time your taste buds change to become used to the natural flavors of food rather than the artificial flavorings you eat at the moment.

Fruits And Vegetables

Fruits and vegetables are high in fiber, vitamin C and anti-oxidants. They are also full of various micro-nutrients that your body really needs in order to repair and maintain itself. Fresh fruits and vegetables are by far the best, but canned or frozen versions are useful for their longer shelf life. Make sure though that any canned versions do not have added sugar or salt as that negates much of the benefit of the product.

Fruits and vegetables help to reduce your risk of heart disease and cancers so are really very beneficial for you.

Popular fruits and vegetables eaten on this diet includes zucchini, carrots, spinach, broccoli, onions, leeks, cabbage, asparagus, cauliflower, eggplant, bell peppers, squashes, sweet potato, lettuce, garlic and squashes. Fruits such as lemons, limes, oranges, apples, pears, melons, cherries, plums, bananas, olives, figs and pineapples are also very popular.

Fruit juice is great, though watch for additives. For the best fruit juices you should make your own but that's another book entirely!

Cereals

Whole grain cereals are full of fiber, vitamins, minerals, protein and complex carbohydrates. These help to reduce the risk of cancer and heart disease as well as reduce bowel problems and lower cholesterol.

Some people do have an intolerance to gluten, in which case these are not suited to you; use some of the alternatives on the market.

Popular cereals include oats, millet, wheat, barley, corn and brown rice which can be found in cereals, muesli, porridge, wholemeal bread, wholemeal pasta, polenta, couscous and more.

Legumes

These grow in pods and are typically high in vitamin B and C as well as fiber, protein and carbohydrates. They are proven to help reduce the risk of heart disease.

Peas, peanuts, chickpeas, beans and lentils are all very good for you and you can find them in cans (low sodium versions) and use them to make soups, stews or even dips such as hummus.

Seafood

Seafood is very good for you and is very high on protein whilst being low in fat. It provides you with many of the essential vitamins and minerals that your body requires. Oily fish are high in Omega-3 oils as well as vitamins A and D whilst whole fish contain phosphorus and calcium. Shellfish are a good source of various trace minerals too. Increasing the amount of these in your diet whilst reducing the amount of red meat will help to protect your heart and reduce the risk of heart disease.

Whole fish such as sardines, pilchards, anchovies and whitebait are all great on this diet as are oily fish such as herring, trout, tuna, mackerel and salmon. Other fish that are commonly eaten include cod, plaice, haddock, halibut, sea bass, whiting, mullet, squid, mussels, crab, prawns and lobster.

Some fish can contain low levels of pollutants from the sea and anyone who is pregnant or trying for a baby needs to avoid certain types of fish.

Foods To Be Carefully Measured

As with any foods, eating too much can result in a health risk if consumed in excess. When cooking foods in this diet you use unsaturated oils instead of saturated animals fats like lard and butter. If you are covering your meals with cheese or cream based sauces then you are adding unhealthy saturated fat to your food.

Instead of using a lot of cheese, use a smaller amount of a stronger cheese or roast your vegetables in olive oil. Unbuttered, wholemeal bread makes for a great and healthy way to mop up juice and sauce on a plate.

Fast foods really need to be avoided as they are full of salt, saturated fats and often trans fats too. These are really bad for you and studies have repeatedly shown that fast food is pretty dangerous stuff!

The Mediterranean Diet has a similar total fat content to the Western diet, though the former is full of mono-unsaturated fats which are healthy and good for you. The Western diet is usually full of saturated fats which clog your arteries up.

Fats

The focus in the Mediterranean Diet is on mono-unsaturated oils which will come from Olive oil or the cheaper alternative, rapeseed oil. Mono-unsaturated oils can be found in nuts, seeds and avocados as well as olives. You can eat whole olives, though again check what they are packaged in.

Olive oil is really very good for you because it contains many essential fatty acids and helps you to absorb vitamins. Olive oil does not degrade in to toxic components when it is heated. It will protect you from heart disease, certain cancers and help to reduce your blood pressure.

However, you do need to be careful as olive oil is high in calories so you can find you put on weight if you use too much. It is best to limit the amount of olive oil you use if you want to lose weight.

Lean White Meat

This is generally chicken but can be turkey and any other poultry. Chicken fast food and processed pies are generally high in saturated animal fats and so do not count as lean white meat.

If you remove the skin then lean white meat is full of protein and vitamins, including B12 which is very important to your health. Eating too much of this can result in you consuming too much saturated fat which is bad for you and can contribute to weight gain. However, in moderation white meat is full of essential minerals and nutrients which are vital to the health of your body.

Nuts And Seeds

Nuts and seeds are part of the Mediterranean Diet and are full of minerals and vitamins as well as protein and fiber. They also contain the healthy unsaturated fats that your body needs as well as plenty of calories so try not to eat too many each day as it will hinder weight loss.

All nuts are eaten unsalted and include walnuts, cashew nuts, Brazil nuts, almonds and chestnuts. Seeds include pumpkin, sesame, poppy, linseed and sunflower; all of which should be unsalted and raw.

Seeds make for a great addition to bread and you can even add nuts to some breads and cakes.

Nuts and seeds will help to protect you against heart disease, diabetes and reduce your cholesterol levels. They also make for a great snack with some dried fruit instead of cookies or cakes.

Wine

Red wine is very good for you and is high in anti-oxidants and other beneficial components. It is high in calories though so will contribute to weight gain if you drink too much. Two or three glasses a day will be plenty when drunk with a meal and pregnant women should avoid alcohol completely.

Red wine is often used in cooking and, when combined with the Mediterranean Diet, provides a high level of protection against heart disease.

Restricted Foods

The foods discussed in this section are high in essential nutrients but if consumed in excess can carry health risks.

Dairy Produce

Dairy produce includes cheese, cream, butter, yogurt, milk, fromage frais, creamy curries, creamy desserts and creamy sauces.

Whilst dairy is high in protein, calcium, vitamin B12 and vitamin A they can also be high in the bad animal fats. Cream and butter are particularly high in fat and are worth avoiding as much as possible. Butter made with olive oil is better but still can still contain the animal fats.

Feta cheese, mozzarella and cottage cheese are lower in saturated fats. Ricotta cheese is very high in fat and you can get reduced fat cheeses. Be aware that some dairy products have salt added to them.

Whilst dairy is a good source of calcium, too much can increase your risk of heart disease and cholesterol levels. Low or no fat dairy produce will reduce your fat intake which is much healthier.

Red Meat

Red meat such as beef, pork and lamb, often eat in fast food, sausages and pies is very high in protein and vitamins, including the vital B12 as well as containing high levels of iron. Lean meat is much better for you but even that can contain high levels of saturated animal fat.

Whilst there are many nutrients in red meat, most of them can be gained from white meat, seafood and vegetables which reduces the risks associated with red meat. Too much red meat will increase your risk of heart disease and increases your cholesterol levels.

You could save your red meat for special occasions such as a special Sunday meal. You could weigh out portions of red meat and then divide it up and use it sparingly in rice and pasta dishes throughout the week.

Potatoes

Potatoes are found in all sorts of pies and processed foods and are a good source of energy. The contain fiber, vitamin C, B vitamins and potassium as well as being high in starch which your body rapidly converts to glucose. However, these high starch levels can increase your risk of type 2 diabetes. One of the main issues with potatoes comes from how they are prepared – often they are cooked in fats and heavily salted.

Desserts

Most processed desserts have absolutely no nutritional value though they taste nice! They can be very high in sugar and saturated fats as well as contained a lot of calories which will increase your waistline.

Milk based desserts will contain some calcium and dark chocolate contains anti-oxidants. Sweet foods like this damage your teeth, increase your risk of heart disease and type 2 diabetes as well as contribute to obesity.

Reduce your reliance on these sweet desserts and relegate them to an occasional treat rather than a daily meal. A good alternative is fresh fruit with yogurt which is deliciously sweet and very good for you!

You can see there is a lot you can eat and a lot to avoid, but the foods you avoid are all for your benefit as they are going to make you healthier and reduce your risk of diseases.

THE IMPORTANCE OF WINE IN THIS DIET

Wine is a very important part of the Mediterranean Diet and it is drunk daily by many people around this sea. The difference is that it is drank socially with food and not to excess. A lot of research is underway into red wine and it is being shown that in moderation it is extremely beneficial for your health. You may be sad to know that other alcoholic drinks do not have the same health benefits.

If you do not like red wine then grape juice made from purple or Concord grapes will provide very similar benefits, but without the alcohol.

Red wine is jam packed full of useful nutrients that help keep you healthy and strong; it really is the nectar of the gods in many respects!

Rioja wine is made from Tempranillo grapes which, like many other red grapes, have an effect on reducing your cholesterol levels. According to a study, people with high cholesterol saw a 12% drop in their LDL or bad cholesterol levels when they took a supplement based on red wine. This means that the LDL is not being deposited on your arterial walls and furring them up, which leads to an increase in blood pressure and in the worst cases, heart attacks.

Red wine contains polyphenols which are antioxidants which have been shown to keep your blood vessels flexible and further reduce the risk of clotting in your arteries.

The skin of a red grape is the best source of resveratrol, which is another antioxidant found in red wine. This antioxidant is the focus of a lot of scientific research because of its health benefits. One benefits of resveratrol is that it appears to help diabetics regular their blood sugar levels! In a study, diabetics who took a 250mg resveratrol supplement daily for three months enjoyed a lower blood glucose level than those that were not taking the supplement. Those who took the supplement also had lower cholesterol levels and a lower systolic blood pressure. It appears that resveratrol stimulates insulin secretion or activates a protein which regulates your insulin and glucose sensitivity.

Resveratrol also has toher benefits in that it appears to assist in keeping your memory sharp. It hampers the formation of the beta-amyloid protein, which is found in the brains of Alzheimer's suffers.

The benefits of red wine do not just stop there because it also appears that the antioxidants found in red wine help keep you well and healthy! In a 2010 study at five Spanish universities, it was found that those people who drank 2 glasses of red wine a night were 40% less likely to get the common cold! The antioxidants in red wine help to fight infection and protect your cells from free radicals.

Even drinking a single glass of red wine just three or four times a week has an effect against cancer cells. It appears that it starves nascent cancer cells. When human cancer cells were dosed with resveratrol it inhibited the actions of a key cancer feeding protein.

When you consume wine your body converts the resveratrol into piceatannol which is helpful in weight loss as it prevents the growth of fat cells, according to lab tests. Piceatannol binds itself to insulin receptors in fat cells which prevent the cells from maturing and growing.

You need to be careful to not cross the line from drinking for your health to drinking too much. Whilst drinking red wine in moderation is good for you, too much is not and will help you gain weight. Too much wine is linked to high blood pressure and heart disease so make sure you moderate your intake! Experts recommend that a woman has one four ounce glass per day and a man has one or two.

If you already suffer from conditions such as high blood pressure, pancreatitis, liver disease, heart problems or high triglycerides then you need to be very careful about drinking red wine as it could make your condition worse. You need to check with your medical professional first to ensure it is safe for you to do so. If you take aspirin regularly for your heart then you will also need to speak to a health care professional first.

Wine is an important part of the Mediterranean lifestyle and it is not drunk to excess, unlike in the west where many people regularly drink too much. Wine forms a part of their social life and is often drunk (in moderation) whilst socializing or during the meal. Other forms of alcohol are not good for you and do not carry the associated health benefits so you need to stick to red wine or red grape juice to get these healthy benefits.

LOOSING WEIGHT BY EATING MEDITERRANEAN

There are many health benefits associated with the Mediterranean Diet and those alone are going to be worth making the shift. However, it can be used to lose weight as well. Earlier on when we were discussing the different foods you can eat and those you should avoid we mentioned some foods which are high in calories and should not be eaten too frequently.

In general the Mediterranean Diet is lower in calories whilst being higher in nutrients, fiber and anti-oxidants. Ensuring you monitor your intake of high calorie foods such as olive oil, bread, meat and nuts will help you to lose weight but the simple act of cutting out the heavily processed, high calorie foods you were consuming will make a huge difference too.

Whilst the daily recommended calorie intake for a man is 2500kcal and 2000kcal for a woman, it is very easy to consume that in a single meal meaning many people can eat two or three times this recommended amount without even thinking about it! This makes it very easy for you to put on weight which will start to drop off when you make the move to the Mediterranean diet, though really keep an eye on your calorie intake.

It can help you to manage your hunger if you divide your food into four or five meals for the day with healthy snacks in between, if required. This can help with digestion and helps you to feel full, which reduces your temptation to snack on unhealthy foods.

Wholemeal pasta is a key component in the Mediterranean Diet and helps you to feel full for longer. Eating this as a part of your meals with plenty of vegetables and a drizzle of olive oil is a very good meal for you. This will provide you with plenty of nutrients, as much if not more than a three course meal, whilst being significantly lower in calories.

Have some bread with your meal, and this is the traditional Italian breads which are not made with butter or unhealthy oils. These or multi-grain breads are ideal as they can help you to feel full.

Olive oil should be your only choice of fat when working to lose weight. It helps with the digestion of other fats and is very beneficial to your health.

Red meat consumption should be minimized when losing weight as it is high in both calories and fat. Chicken, pork, turkey and rabbit are preferred because they have the same nutritional benefits but a lot less fat.

Fish is another good thing to eat to help you lose weight. Fish such as sardines and anchovies are high in nutrition whilst low in fat.

Fruits and vegetables are important too and they can be eaten raw or with pasta, fish or meat. These are high in the fiber and minerals that your body needs to thrive and look after itself.

Weight loss is actually quite pleasurable on the Mediterranean Diet because of the variety of foods your can eat. It is very good for you and filling yet is not as calorie dense as some of the Western meals. A single meal from a fast food restaurant could represent most of your daily calorie intake so eating these healthy, lower calorie meals often results in weight loss. The best thing is though is as you are losing weight so you are looking after your health too.

7 DAY MEDITERRANEAN DIET PLAN

A lot of books will give you a list of foods to eat and tell you exactly what you need to follow over the next week to get in to the Mediterranean Diet. The problem I always have with this is that there is usually a few dishes I do not like or have things in I cannot get hold of, which makes the plan hard to follow.

In this book we are going to do things slightly differently and instead of giving you a rigid structure to follow I will share with you a more flexible framework and help you to create your own week long plan that you will enjoy following. By making it easy for you like this you are more likely to follow the plan and realize the many benefits of this eating program!

This way you are more likely to stick to the diet because you are eating foods that you enjoy and can work the diet around your lifestyle. If you get home from work late, spending two hours cooking an evening meal may well be completely impractical for you. This will invariably lead to snacking and calling for takeout because you are tired and not in the mood to prepare a meal.

Many of the meals though in this book can be prepared in advance and frozen. This is my favorite way of preparing food which means that all I need to do is heat up the food and I have a healthy meal when I need it. For someone who works full time, this can be a simple way to follow the diet.

Creating your own seven day Mediterranean eating program is remarkably simple to do. Just follow these steps:

- Pick five to seven breakfasts.
- Pick five to seven lunches.
- Pick five to seven dinners.
- Pick five to seven desserts.
- Pick three or four breads.
- Pick around a dozen or so snacks.
- Pick two or three bottles of good quality red wine.

Then organize these into a plan for the next week based on a breakfast, lunch, dinner and dessert each day plus one loaf of bread for every two days and a bottle of wine to last two or three days! Work this plan out based on your schedule for the week. For example, if you know you are going to be late home one night then use leftovers from the previous night or choose a quick dish.

This way you have your own seven day eating plan that is easy for you to stick to, works for your lifestyle and has foods your love in it! It is simple to do and much better than trying to stick to an eating program that just is not practical for you.

MEDITERRANEAN DIET TIPS

The Mediterranean Diet is pretty easy to follow once you get the hang of it, but this chapter is designed to help you really get to grips with the diet and make the most of it.

Extra Virgin Olive Oil Is Your One Fat

This fat has been called "liquid gold" by Homer and "the great therapeutic" by Hippocrates, the father of modern medicine. It is an oil which has significant health benefits and just by replacing many of the other fats used in the Western diet with Olive oil it could make a major difference in the health of the population.

Olive oil has a very high percentage of oleic acid which is a mono-unsaturated fatty acid proven to protect your heart. It also contains polyphenols which are anti-oxidants that prevent inflammation and stops oxidation (damage) to your cells. Olive oil is also very high in vitamin E which is another vitamin with anti-oxidant properties.

Always make sure you have a bottle of extra virgin olive oil in your kitchen and use it when grilling fish or vegetables. It can be used to make a vinaigrette dressing that is delicious on salads and can be used on almost anything you eat! It even makes a good alternative to butter for your bread. It is definitely a major, must have part of the Mediterranean Diet.

Eat Greens And Colorful Vegetables With Every Meal

Mediterranean food is renowned for its color with juicy red tomatoes, dark green spinach and crunch yellow and orange bell peppers. All of these help to heal your body and are considered nature's medicine chest. Farmer's markets are great sources of fresh produce at affordable prices. They are high in vitamins and minerals as well as polyphenols.

With your dinner and lunch have a fresh green salad dressed with extra virgin olive oil or lemon juice. This is a healthy addition to your diet and will ensure you get plenty of the vital vitamins.

My personal favourite is to roast a selection of vegetables with a drizzle of extra virgin olive oil. These are great with pasta or even in a wrap with pesto sauce.

Fruit Is Important

A good variety of food is excellent for your heart and health. Mediterranean fruits such as figs, pomegranate, lemons and oranges are packed full of vitamins that are good for you.

Other fruits such as kiwi, apples, melons and bananas should be included too as they are delicious and also good for you.

Berries make a great breakfast and a good dessert in the evening with some yogurt. Dried fruits such as cranberries, currants and apricots go well in a lunchtime salad and are high in anti-oxidants!

Fruit is very good for you, being very healthy and sweet. Often for someone who is craving sweet foods, a nice bowl of fruit is ideal and will satisfy that need.

Eat Lentils Or Legumes Ever Day

Lentils have been at the receiving end of many a joke since they became popular with vegetarians but they are an essential part of the Mediterranean diet. Lentils are absolutely loaded with anti-oxidants, fiber, protein, iron, minerals and vitamins and best of all are very cheap and easily available! They are a superb food to eat that will ensure a healthy heart.

You can get your legumes by dipping raw vegetables in to hummus, adding kidney beans or chickpeas (from a can is fine) to a salad and eating soups based on legumes such as split pea, black bean, lentil, minestrone and so on.

Fish Is Eaten Regularly

Fish has long been known to be extremely good for you and in Greenland the native population had no incidences of heart disease; all put down to a diet high in seafood!

Fish oil is a major component of the Mediterranean Diet and it is high in Omega-3 fatty acids, which are very good for your health. Rather than eating red meat, choose fish instead. You can buy fresh fish from your supermarket though make sure it smells fresh (i.e. not fishy). You can then cut it up into servings, wrap it and freeze any excess.

Salmon and tuna are excellent fish to eat and can often be found when you are eating out, making a healthy way of sticking to your diet. If you have it grilled and dressed with a squeeze of lemon juice then it is perfect for the Mediterranean Diet.

Eat Walnuts

Walnuts are contribute a lot to the health benefits of the Mediterranean Diet because they are high in alpha-linolenic acid (ALA) which is an omega-3 fatty acid which is only found in plants.

Walnuts can easily be introduced in to your diet and used either as a snack or included in salads or other meals. You can sprinkle some crushed walnuts with Greek yogurt and honey for a quick and healthy dessert. Walnuts can be candied with brown sugar, sprinkled on salads or just eaten raw, depending on your preference.

Eat Whole Grains

The Mediterranean diet does not involve processed grains, which are such a staple part of the Western diet. When you eat whole grains you get the nutrition from all three parts of the grain (bran, endosperm and germ), much of which is stripped out in our manufacturing processes.

Ideally you want three servings of whole grains every day and popcorn does count and makes a great snack if you make it yourself. A great seasoning is a few sprays of olive oil plus some parmesan cheese or brown sugar, depending on your preference.

Oatmeal makes for a really healthy breakfast that keeps you feeling full for longer. Steel cut oatmeal is the best for you as it is high in beta-glucan and you can make a large batch of it then heat it up every morning. Whole grain breads are your bread of choice and whole grain pasta is also the best option.

Drink Red Wine

Red wine, as you know, is very important to your health on the Mediterranean diet, being full of powerful, healthy giving antioxidants. Avoid white wine as red has ten times more antioxidants! A glass or two a night is enough, you do not need any more as drinking to excess causes more harm than good. If you do not want to drink wine then red grape juice will have the same beneficial effect without the alcohol.

Dark Chocolate Is Good For You!

Dark chocolate is proving to have some surprising health benefits for your heart and blood vessels! Either eat raw dark chocolate or make a home-made hot chocolate by mixing two spoons of natural, unsweetened, dark chocolate cocoa powder with some sweetener and milk. Heat it up and you have a decadent but healthy drink! Use dark chocolate in your cooking as unsweetened, natural cocoa powder has a high concentration of antioxidants and is low in calories and sugar.

Exercise Is Vital

In the Mediterranean people are more active than they are in the West. Instead of relying on their car for everything they will walk, garden and take other physical exercise. It is important for you to take moderate exercise such as walking, swimming or other exercise you like. Try to integrate it in to your life so instead of driving to the shop for your newspaper, walk instead. Ideally you want a minimum of 30 minutes physical activity every day, though more moderate exercise will not cause you any harm.

These tips will help make the Mediterranean diet much easier for you to follow and help you benefit from it. This diet has a huge amount of benefits and when you integrate all of it in to your life you will be shocked at the difference it makes to your life!

ENDNOTE

The Mediterranean Diet is not nearly as complex as you may think and if more people followed this way of eating then there would be far fewer incidents of serious disease in the west. With the areas that naturally follow this diet enjoy long, healthy lives without serious illness, this is a diet that everyone should be considering eating.

This diet does require some changes in that way you approach food, but they are relatively minor changes for significant benefits. When you consider how much you can reduce your risk of serious illness just by changing what you eat as well as hear some of the miracle stories associated with this diet you will soon realize why more people need to be eating in this way.

By removing processed foods that are high in unhealthy fats, chemicals and sugars and replacing them with more natural foods you are giving your body the vitamins and minerals it needs in order to work at peak efficiency and repair itself. You will be surprised at the difference in your health after you have been following this diet even for just a few weeks.

Like any diet, the Mediterranean Diet works best when combined with exercise because this will help you to be even healthier and lose weight, if that is one of your goals. Don't worry, you don't have to become a gym bunny, just some moderate exercise for around 30 minutes a day is enough to have significant health benefits. This can be as simple as taking a walk at lunchtime or using the stairs throughout the day instead of elevators.

There are a lot of different types of food you can eat, and this diet does not have to be boring at all! You can make this diet very varied and still enjoy many of the foods that you enjoy without having to feel that you are going without or struggling to find nice food to eat.

This book will have given you all the guidance you need in getting started on the Mediterranean diet and eating in this health giving way. There are plenty of recipes and plenty of ideas for sticking to this diet, which is the problem many people face when following any diet.

Take the time to create your own seven day eating program from the information in this book and then follow this diet for a week. In a week's time, see how you are feeling and how you have enjoyed the diet! You can then make another plan, add in some more recipes and continue to enjoy the diet. Give it a few weeks and you will be seeing a difference in your health as well as your waistline. I started following this diet and within two weeks was being asked by people what I was taking as the lines around my eyes were disappearing and I was apparently looking younger ever week! People were convinced I had discovered a miracle age cream and were somewhat surprised that it was down to diet. Many of my friends now follow this diet, at least 75% of the time and are also enjoying the benefits from it.

One of the best things about the Mediterranean Diet is that it still allows you to go out for meals. Sure, you can go to a Greek, Lebanese or Italian restaurant and get 'authentic' cuisine, which is an obvious first choice to ensure you stick to the diet. However, many other restaurants will serve at least one Italian or Mediterranean style dish that, if not 100% compatible with your diet, is mostly suitable for this diet.

With some carefully planning, some preparation in advance and some freezing you can easily follow this diet, no matter how busy you are. It has a massive amount of benefits for your health and your waistline and you really owe it to yourself to follow this diet and enjoy living a long, healthy life!

Printed in Great Britain
by Amazon